Springer Series on Rehabilitation

Myron G. Eisenberg, PhD, Series Editor
Veterans Affairs Medical Center, Hampton, VA
Thomas E. Backer, PhD, Consulting Editor
Human Interaction Research Institute, Los Angeles, CA

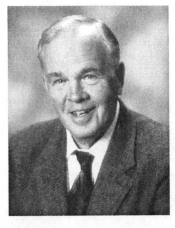

Paul W. Power, ScD, CRC, is an Emeritus Professor of Counseling, University of Maryland. Dr. Power is the author of numerous articles, books, and book chapters on the topic of the family and disability. His speeches and workshops, on both national and international levels, have also focused on the roles of the family on the treatment and rehabilitation process. Specifically, he has co-authored and co-edited with Arthur dell Orto: *Brain Injury and the Family: A Life and Living Perspective* (2000), *The Role of the Family in the Rehabilitation of the Physically Disabled* (1980), and *Family Interventions Throughout Chronic Illness and Disability* (Springer, 1988).

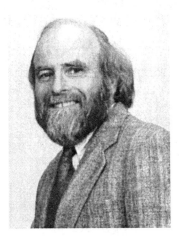

Arthur E. Dell Orto, PhD, CRC, is Professor and Program Director of Rehabilitation Counseling in the Department of Rehabilitation Sciences, Sargent College of Health and Rehabilitation Sciences at Boston University and is the Associate Executive Director of Boston University's Center for Psychiatric Rehabilitation.

He was awarded a B.A. in psychology in 1966 and M.A. in rehabilitation counseling in 1968 from Seton Hall University. He received a Ph.D. in Counseling and Rehabilitation from Michigan State University in 1970. Dr. Dell Orto is a licensed psychologist and a Certified Rehabilitation Counselor whose academic and clinical interests relate to the role of the family in the treatment and rehabilitation process.

Dr. Dell Orto has given many presentations and workshops focusing on the needs of families living with illness and disability.

He has co-authored and co-edited with Paul Power: *The Resilient Family* (2003), *Brain Injury and the Family* (2000); *Head Injury and the Family: A Life and Living Approach* (1994): Awarded Pyramid of Distinction and an Award of Excellence by the New England Association of the American Medical Writers; *Illness and Disability: Family Interventions Throughout the Life Span* (Springer, 1988); *Role of the Family in the Rehabilitation of the Physically Disabled* (1980). He has also co-edited the following books: *The Encyclopedia of Disability and Rehabilitation* (1995): Awarded an "Excellence in Media Award" by The National Rehabilitation Association; *The Psychological and Social Impact of Disability* (Springer, 1999 & 1991), *The Psychological and Social Impact of Physical Disability* (Springer, 1984 & 1977); and *Group Counseling and Physical Disability* (1979).

Families Living With Chronic Illness and Disability

Interventions, Challenges, and Opportunities

Paul W. Power, ScD, CRC
Arthur E. Dell Orto, PhD, CRC

 Springer Publishing Company

Springer Publishing Company, Inc.
536 Broadway
New York, NY 10012-3955

Acquisitions Editor: Helvi Gold
Production Editor: Janice Stangel
Cover design by Joanne Honigman

04 05 06 07 08 / 5 4 3 2 1

Library of Congress Cataloging-in-Publication Data

Families living with chronic illness and disability : interventions, challenges, and opportunities / Paul W. Power & Arthur E. Dell Orto.—1st ed.
    p. cm. — (Springer series on rehabilitation)
  Includes bibliographical references and index.
  ISNB 0-8261-5581-2
  1. Chronically ill—Family relationships. 2. People with disabilities—Family relationships. 3. Chronically ill—Rehabilitation. 4. People with disabilities—Rehabilitation.
  I. Dell Orto, Arthur E., 1943- II. Title. III. Series.
RC108.P69 2004
362.196'044—dc22   2004011469

Printed in the United States of America by Integrated Book Technology.

To Barbara Ann Power, loving wife and trusted friend, whose editorial and computer skills, and self-sacrifice and patience were all responsible to bring this book to completion.

Contents

Preface

This book is a needed, practical, supportive response to the complex challenges that families face when a family member has a chronic illness or severe disability. With the onset of a disabling condition in one of its members, the entire family usually begins a journey filled with disappointment, pervasive pain and anger, as well as joy, love, and hope. As the family attempts to adapt to the given medical situation, and bears the day by day burden of coping, factors within the family influence the medical and emotional functioning of the person with the chronic illness or severe disability. The family may also become a major source of assistance to an individual's rehabilitation or adjustment, or a significant stumbling block to the attainment of treatment goals.

Although there has been an explosion of research related to illness and disability, there is still little attention paid to how the family can become a helping resource for the family member's adjustment to illness and disability—and eventual rehabilitation. The family can make a difference and play an important role at every stage of the illness or disability, though too often the total rehabilitation treatment efforts have only focused on helping the patient. To assist the family in playing this partnering role, a greater focus during intervention efforts must be placed on their emotional and behavioral response to the medical situation, on understanding what the family member who is seriously ill or disabled is emotionally experiencing, and on the relevant intergenerational life experiences, and current and future family needs.

This book discusses all of the issues cited above and also provides distinctive models of family assessment and family intervention. Several of the chapters are unique in their discussion since they bring together existing literature and provide the authors' viewpoints on how this research is applicable to families who are characterized by increased vulnerabilities, ongoing losses, and actual or potential gains. With chapters focusing on "Working with Health Professionals," and "Perspectives on Illness and Disability," the reader can gain different insights on how to either create enhanced opportunities to offering family assistance to members who are severely ill or disabled, or to develop smoother, more negotiable pathways to appropriate family life adjustment.

This book is a combination of original material and personal statements by individuals experiencing the chronic illness or severe disability. This material is supplemented by structured experiential exercises and discussion questions related to the themes of each chapter. The original material is presented as a reflection of thoughts based on our professional and personal experiences, prior publications (Power & Dell Orto, 2003: Dell Orto & Power, 1994, 2000; Power, Dell Orto, & Gibbons, 1988; Power & Dell Orto, 1980), and interpretations of the works of others. The unique personal statements put into thought-provoking perspective the issues that are relevant to treatment, family adaptation, quality of life, and family survival. These statements represent special contributions by our friends and establish a personalized framework for the book material. They give reality to the theoretical material contained in the chapter. The structured experiential tasks (SET) are designed to facilitate the reader's exploration of issues that are the major themes of each chapter.

For helping families to manage an intense medical event, we believe that a family-oriented life and living perspective should be combined with a family intervention philosophy that not only includes an acknowledgment of the adverse effects of the illness and disability, but also emphasizes an affirmation approach to family struggles and opportunities. This orientation and philosophy is a foundation for building a viable treatment and rehabilitation process that supports and encourages families to become a resource for themselves and their family members during the sometimes long adaptive journey.

The authors are also aware that for many families, chronic illness and disability is often in addition to other stressors and problems. Some families or individual family members, consequently, may not be willing or able to engage in a demanding involvement with the individual who is seriously ill or disabled, especially when the outcome is often unknown. It is from this perspective, as well as from the realization that many family members are eager to assume challenging responsibilities, that this book will assist the reader to discover ways to involve the family in the ill or disabled person's rehabilitation. Also, by understanding the authors' responses to the following questions, readers can gain new insights into the issues associated with both this involvement and the families' own adjustment process:

- How does the family influence, impede, or facilitate the adjustment of a family member who is living with a chronic disease or severe disability?

- What are the general limitations and resources, as well as possible limitations and resources of the family, during the treatment and rehabilitation process?
- How can health and human care providers assist families in maintaining balance in their lives as well as maintain a reasonable quality of life?

The intended audience for this book includes health, allied health, and other professionals whose work responsibilities will bring them in contact with families as they pursue their interventions with the identified patient, for example, physicians, nurses, rehabilitation counselors, social workers, psychologists, family advocates, physical and occupational therapists, clergy, peer counselors, and speech pathologists.

It is also intended for those still in training within these allied health professions. In the estimation of the authors, all of these people have a unique opportunity to understand and appreciate family dynamics when severe disability and chronic disease affect the family members, to provide support for the family, and to share information about effective coping strategies and community resources.

Today, and for the foreseeable future, many persons with a severe disability or chronic disease and their families may be cast adrift in a sea of confusing uncertainty and hope often fueled by desperation. While many problems related to living with and in spite of an intense medical event have been managed or solved at the beginning of this new millennium, the bottom line is that for many families there is still the ever-present need of further managing a vulnerable quality of life. These needs and challenges are recognized and discussed in this book, while emphasizing the theme that a realistic life and living perspective is based upon a vision of hope for all involved.

Paul W. Power
Arthur E. Dell Orto

Acknowledgments

This book is the collective effort of many persons. We would like to thank those men and women who are living the family experience with disability, are role models, and who have contributed their personal stories which have not only enriched this book, but have also brought reality to the theoretical material presented in this volume. Special mention is given to Helvi Gold, who initially encouraged this project and then provided valuable, continued support to us, and to Janice Stangel for her editorial assistance and patience. Their professional contributions have provided insights, wisdom, and understanding.

Part I

Family Dynamics in Illness and Disability

O ne of the main tenets of this book is that the family is frequently a potent influence in shaping the way a person adjusts to an illness or disability (Jaffe, 1978; Dell Orto & Power, 2000). A family-focused approach is likely to maximize intervention effectiveness, whether or not other family members are directly involved in the health-related behaviors that the intervention is designed to change (Weihs, Fisher & Baird, 2002). The starting point or continuation of the long journey for the family and its member who are living with illness and disability is to identify those resources that can make a difference between successful coping or prolonged periods of desperation and utter disappointment. During treatment and rehabilitation families must learn to identify which bridges to cross, which to burn, which to avoid, which to modify, and which to build (Rocchio, 1998a).

The four chapters in this section focus on the many changes that occur in family life. These changes are precursors to understanding both the needs of family members while living the illness or disability experience, and what intervention strategies can be useful for the family's own adjustment and its ability to assist the member who is ill or disabled. With disability and the onset of illness in either an adult or child, family members will usually have emotional and behavior changes, and consequently other changes are created in the family, including a new meaning for family life. Unfortunately, families are forced to be reactive to illness and disability because they may not have based their life perspective on a frame of reference that includes the reality of the unexpected. Who expected September 11th? Who is prepared for a September12th? Anything can happen to anyone. What we expect to happen, might happen, and what we do not expect to happen, often will.

Chapter 1, in identifying the many perspectives needed to embrace an insightful understanding of illness and disability, provides a context and a philosophy for assisting a family both to achieve an appropriate quality of life following the advent of an intense medical situation, and for helping the family become an instrumental, positive influence on the family member during treatment and rehabilitation. It emphasizes the authors' belief that disability is a family affair. Chapters two and three focus on the child and adult, respectively, and discuss the family member's needs that cry out for a timely response, and the emotions that can be important factors for considering a person's life adjustment. These varied emotions and coping styles may also become inhibitors from assisting the ill or disabled member from attaining stabilizing rehabilitation goals. Collectively, moreover, the family has distinctive responses to the medical event. Similar to the material presented in the previous chapters, chapter four discusses these reactions and identifies the determinants of family reactions and the themes of the family's responses. All of these chapters lay the foundation for the flexible, targeted interventions detailed in Part II.

The personal statements of Janet, Celia, Alina, and Ted and his mother show how individual reactions to a chronic illness or severe disability shape family life and become opportunities for discovering a new, and perhaps fulfilling, meaning to life and living. They also accentuate the truth that most families are vulnerable because they live their lives based upon untested belief systems. Each statement brings home the launching truth that all families should have options and opportunities to access those resources that can minimize unnecessary frustrations and disappointments, and facilitate stabilization, growth, and resilience.

REFERENCES

Dell Orto, A. E. & Power, P. W. (2000). *Brain injury and the family*, 2nd Ed. Boca Raton: CRC Press.

Jaffe, D. T. (1978). The role of family therapy in treating physical illness. *Hospital and Community Psychiatry, 29*, 170–174.

Rocchio, C. (1998a). The unvarnished truth: There is no cure for brain injury. *Family News and Views, Brain Injury Association, 2*(4), 34–35.

Weihs, K., Fisher, L., & Baird, M. (2002). Families, health, and behavior: A section of the commissioned report by the Committee of Hhealth and Behavior: Research, practice, and policy. *Families, Systems & Health, 20*(1), 17–46.

1

Perspectives on Illness and Disability

All families have dreams. They dream that there will be a bright future for them and their family, that their children will be successful, and that health and happiness will be the rule rather than the exception. However, as the extraordinary life-altering events of September 11, 2001 illustrate, in an instant anyone's world can be shattered or transformed. While the dramatic pictures of this tragedy are etched into the minds and souls of all who bore witness to these events, many families and individuals are living with similar life-altering realities related to loss and change, often consequent to illness and disability. In effect their world has been affected and has collapsed. With this dramatic change a new reality and new set of options have emerged. The causes are different but there is a common ground of personal and familial transformations that are consequent to life and living, illness and disability, loss and change. McDaniel, Hepworth, and Doherty (1999) crystallized this point related to illness when they stated:

> Today, in the narrative of every human life and every family, illness remains a prominent character. Even if so far we have avoided serious illness ourselves, we cannot escape its reach into our family lives and our friendship circles. Illness brings us closer to one another in care giving, and it separates us through disability and death. It moves us to make sense of our lives and it creates confusion and doubt. It inspires courage and fear, hope and despair, and serenity and anxiety. From childhood onward, our personal and family experiences of illness shape us as surely as the food we eat and the love or rejection we experience (p. 2).

This chapter will identify several perspectives that will frame the subsequent chapters in this book. These perspectives are both realities emerging from the family experience of living with a chronic illness or severe disability, and foundational blocks upon which is established a family infrastructure. This infrastructure can provide support when confronted with family loss and disruption. There is an interaction between the realities and the building blocks, because understanding challenges, stress, change, and health care relationships facilitates the development of a family's foundation for coping. Furthermore, perspectives can be motivational. Understanding an insightful viewpoint may become a stimulus for adaptive action. The perspectives identified below not only embrace all of these factors, but also are reflective of the central topics and themes that will be developed in this book.

THE PERSPECTIVE OF VULNERABILITY

Just as the World Trade Center was considered to be permanent and invulnerable by both those who constructed it and those who worked in it, many families believe that their family and its emotional and physical home can sustain any assault or attack whether it be by a known or some other unexpected or unfamiliar entity. The problem is that illness and disability, as well as many other life challenges, represent more than just an attack or assault. These bio-psycho-social occurrences embrace many other unpredictable "life events" that can affect families at any time, at any place, and often have irreversible as well as undesirable consequences. These events frequently occur when the family is least prepared and often during the initial nightmare of emergency room and medical procedures when families and significant others feel, and often are, vulnerable, abandoned, and are left to fend for themselves while being forced to rely on their meager and faltering resources. The result is that families are put at emotional risk and may feel that they are in an alien health care world where the customs, expectations, and experiences are disconcerting, disorienting, and often perplexing. These emotions are often a result of decisions made in times of crisis. Frequently these decisions are based on desperation, intensified by fear and uncertainty, as well as counterbalanced and energized by hope and optimism. This is a time of great vulnerability and increased need for support, understanding, and hope. It is also a time of unique opportunity, not only to actively respond to what is happening, but also to influence future familial decisions and reactions for generations to come.

Just for a moment consider the fallout from 9/11/01 if most of the 3,027 people who lost their lives had experienced instead a variety of injuries and disabilities and were in need of long-term treatment and rehabilitation This would have created a very different experience and health care scenario for all involved. Rather than the primary focus being on death, loss, and grief, there would have been a great emphasis on hope, treatment, rehabilitation, and restoration. It would be reasonable to assume that most, if not all, of the families who lost family members would be elated if they could have a family member living with a variety of problems rather than cope with the permanent loss of a loved one. However, there are always situations where the quality of life for all involved has been so compromised that some may wish for a different outcome.

While the reactions of the family vary according to the severity of the illness or disability and the subsequent losses, implications, and potential for treatment and rehabilitation, a common denominator for the family is that they, as well as their world, have been changed forever—not necessarily for better or worse, but changed for sure. This change is a result of the initial trauma, the historical and life experiences of the family, and the reality of complex and long-term demands placed on, or anticipated by, the family. In effect, the family has been transformed and moved to a new dimension of life and living for which they are not adequately prepared, and in which the demands are often in excess of the families' resources, supports, perspective, and skills. These extreme conditions and unrealistic expectations can rapidly deplete the most resourceful families and magnify their difficulties which, in turn, may result in intergenerational, interpersonal, emotional, physical, and financial bankruptcy.

One of the major challenges of coping with trauma, loss, or illness and disability is that people are unprepared for the potentially overwhelming reality that can affect their families at any time or place during the life span. Rolland (1994) emphasizes this point when he states that any family can be expected to "hit the wall" when faced with the extraordinary demands of a chronic illness or disability. How many health care providers believe and expect that the family will be able to leap over this "wall" or just stay where they are and get on with their lives? How would they feel if they were faced with similar situations in their own family?

Consequently, most families are vulnerable because they may live their lives based upon untested belief systems and they are often shocked when their beliefs and/or expectations are not validated by reality.

THE PERSPECTIVE OF FAMILY CHALLENGE

For health care professionals who are confronted with a family beginning the long journey of coping with illness and disability, there is the challenge to develop a perspective that assists the family to think clearly, live in a manner that maximizes potential for improvement, contains the impact of non-normative losses, and facilitates the process of appropriate adaptation to change. It is important to consider this perspective when attempting to access and involve the family as a resource during the treatment and rehabilitation process. This is especially so when the family sees ongoing involvement as a process of reliving what has occurred, experiencing more guilt and blame, and harboring the perception of continued burden rather than opportunity. While a sudden event can transform a family, a perspective gained during the severe experience can bring a new dimension to life and living. This is illustrated by the following statements by persons living with the transformation of a family member consequent to the occurrence of illness and disability:

> I will do anything to help my son. Any problem can be solved, any burden can be managed: it is just a matter of perspective. As an engineer I consider problems in need of being solved. Spinal cord injury certainly is a challenging problem.

> My wife is very important to me. Even though she is no longer exactly the same person I married, she was once a great wife and mother and I will never forget that or ever neglect her. I know she would have done the same for me.

> We decided to do the best we can and rely on our friends, family, and faith and practice what we believe in. In some ways our family is closer and stronger after the cancer, as strange as it may sound. It took a major trauma to get all of our attention, and now we focus on what really matters to us—our future together, joy to be had, and peace to be realized.

While these statements differ in emotional content, perspective, and frame of reference, it is important to realize that they are valid frames of reference that indicate where the family has been, where the family is, and where it has to go. Feelings related to frames of reference also capture and indicate the significance of familiar history, the impact of residuals of family interaction, and the role of values and tradition on the willingness of a family to engage in a demanding and often uncertain outcome of the treatment and rehabilitation process. For example, most families believe that illness and disability can and must be prevented, cured, or at least improved, and that people who are ill and disabled should be cared for while having access to quality health care, support, and resources.

However, a critical incident in life and living occurs when individuals and families are "put to the test," and given a chance to practice what they preach or learn what they need to know, and translate beliefs into action. For example, how many people live their lives:

- Believing that their family loves them so much that they will always take care of them regardless of the problems or demands related to illness and disability?
- Making promises that they will never leave each other no matter what challenges, changes, or traumas occur. Some individuals and families make such promises based on experience while others have nothing on which to base their decision.
- Hoping that because they have been self-sacrificing for their children, the children in turn will be equally devoted to them when they are elderly and in need.
- Living a healthy life style as a means to preventing and or eliminating all illness and disability for themselves or their family
- Relying on laws to prevent crimes of violence that could result in personal or familial disability or loss.
- Believing that medical resources will be accessible and improvement possible if enough funding is available and efforts made.

These are beliefs that make people feel good about their humanity and create a frame of reference within which they can interpret the world around them. A major confrontation occurs when expectations are not met, needs are not fulfilled, and dreams are either unattainable or shattered. Families, therefore, are "put to the test," and are given a chance to translate previously held beliefs into expectations that are hopeful as well as realistic. When these beliefs are challenged and tested by the reality of illness or disability, families are often faced with an opportunity to have their beliefs validated or recognize that their beliefs may have been untested myths.

Illness and disability have the potential to challenge familial belief systems because of their complexity, intensity, and multidimensionality. These characteristics force families to not only examine their beliefs and value systems, but also to make major structural adjustments to accommodate the emerging needs of the family member who has experienced the illness and disability and must live with its life-altering consequences. This process is often the cause of individual and familial distress.

THE PERSPECTIVE OF STRESS

Presenting stress in a comprehensive framework, Weihs, Fisher, and Baird (2002) stated:

Chronic disease is a long-term stressor for both the patient and his or her family members. The nature and intensity of this chronic stress has three important determinants. The first is the magnitude of the changes required of the patient and family members in their day-to-day activities and in the way they relate to one another. The changes required to optimize the health and well-being of the patient in the face of the chronic disease vary widely because of the differences in the demand characteristics of each disease and the particular challenges it brings to the family (Rolland, 1994). The second determinant of the level of stress generated by the illness is the capacity of the patient, within the circumstances of the family and their approach to life, to make these changes. The parents, spouses, and other family members are assumed to be the primary source of support, and their ability to meet the needs of the patient is often confounded by the distress that illness generates in other family members (Bailer, Kaufman, Peretz, Manor, Ever-Hadani, & Kaplan-DeNour, 1996; Boss, Caron, Horbal, & Mortimer, 1990). Distressed household members are less able to provide support and may also need assistance (Helgeson, 1994). Finally, the availability of medical assistance and the community resources for support of people with chronic disease can mitigate or exacerbate the stress of illness (p. 9).

Most health and human care systems do not have the same perspective, agendas, or goals as the family and are not primarily designed to meet their changing and emerging needs. This lack of "common ground' often adds to the stress experienced by the family forced to let go of a member, as well as renegotiate a relationship with that individual who is not exactly the person they knew prior to the onset of an illness or disability. In reality, however, nothing in life will be exactly the same and often families must settle for what is realistic compared with the ideal situation.

Discussing adjustment to health loss, Zemzars (1984) said, "a person can never fully return to his or her pre-illness state of health" (p. 44). This does not mean that gains cannot be made or new goals attained or approximated. It does mean, or at least imply, that in many situations all of the losses cannot be fully regained even if this is the driving force and expectation of the family or the health care team. For some families the only goal is to be exactly as they were prior to the onset of the condition.

THE PERSPECTIVE OF FAMILY TRANSFORMATION

A familial transformation consequent to illness and disability and other traumatic life events often occurs when the family is least prepared. The result is that families can be traumatized and put at emotional and physical risk in some hospital and health care environments that may be far from hospitable or caring. From this point of emotional desolation, families are launched into a potentially unending nightmare that may cover weeks, months, years, or a lifetime. This is an extremely lonely and isolating time that demands meaningful as well as frequent support and ongoing stabilization. This should be a point of major importance and concern for health care and human care workers and systems because some families and family members may never be able to move beyond being caught in the vortex of the illness and disability storm and having to live with the ongoing debris from the fallout.

Anyone who has borne witness to the transformation of a life or the reality of the loss of a loved one in a trauma center or hospital can attest to the aloneness and complexity that are often characteristics of these environments. Often they are not family friendly, and by default can intensify pain and suffering rather than alleviate them. At this point, support, caring, relevant interventions, and helpful information are essential in meeting family needs. How families learn about the condition and how well they understand the changes they are undergoing can be factors in reducing or increasing distress.

A PERSPECTIVE FOR HEALTH CARE PROFESSIONALS

While in the process of doing the best job that they can, often under very difficult circumstances, health and human care professionals should keep in mind the profound impact of the information they provide as well as its implications.

Focusing on this process, Garwick, Patterson, Bennet, and Blum (1995) stated:

> The diagnosis experience is a unique and pivotal one for families. Since the time of diagnosis is usually a crisis event for the family, clinicians need to break the news in a way that facilitates the family's adjustment to the news, as well as their ability to care for their child. Whenever possible, clinicians need to plan the setting, assess family background variables (e.g., caregiver's knowledge and experience with chronic illness and disability), and then select the strategies that will help family caregivers hear and understand the information that they need to know. This process of pacing and fitting the information process to the particular needs of the family increases the likelihood that the family caregivers will be able to hear important information (p. 994).

A flawed and often convenient presumption made by some insurance companies, managed care, health care, and rehabilitation systems is that somehow, and at some time, the family is going to be willing and able to bind its resources and respond to role changes, demands, and expectations in order to facilitate the health and emotional care treatment and rehabilitation of a family member. A question to ask is for whose convenience is this? Or is this just a means of shifting responsibility rather than sharing and partnering? It is often easier to abrogate responsibility and expect others to fill the voids of an inadequate system rather than making the needed changes and innovations.

Rocchio (1998) commented on the erosion of financial supports and the shift of expectations to the family:

> Because of managed care constraints, family services that were once a reimbursable expense now have been virtually eliminated. As a result, rehabilitation professionals face a daunting challenge in training families to manage this responsibility themselves. Insurance carriers are all the more eager to bill services under psychiatric benefits, which traditionally have low capitation, than to provide extended neurorehabilitation which will assist family members and individuals with brain injury to attain better outcomes and quality of life (pp. 34–35).

Weihs, Fisher, and Baird (2002) commented on the importance of the family and home environment:

> Because disease management behaviors occur primarily in the home, where they involve and are affected by family members, the social or ecological perspective suggests that interventions to improve disease management should actively address the complex social environment of the home. A family-focused approach is likely to maximize intervention effectiveness, whether or not other family members are directly involved in the health behavior that the intervention is designed to change (p. 10).

An evolving demand for health care professionals, consequently, is to become aware of and responsive to a family's history, as well as to their customary needs now transformed by illness and disability (Weihs, Fisher, & Baird, 2002). With this awareness and responsiveness, these professionals should also come to understand that the success or failure of structural adjustments in the family and its members is often determined by the pre-injury lifestyle of the family. Unfortunately, most families do not prepare themselves for the possibility of any illness or disability that may challenge or erode their beliefs, values, and resources. Families are often forced, consequently, to be reactive to these medical events because they may not have based their own life expectation on a realistic frame of reference related to the total life and living experience. Health care professionals should also gradually realize that most families are vulnerable because they live their lives based upon frequently untested belief systems and are often shocked when their beliefs and expectations are not validated by reality which often relates to the success or failure of medical intervention. If the family is to negotiate successfully this transition from hope to acceptance, then health care professionals should attempt to be on the same wavelength as family members. But some health and human care systems do not have the same agendas or goals as the family and may not be primarily designed to meet the changing and emerging needs of families. Connell and Connell (1995) reinforce this point when they state: "Obstacles to coping and recovery exist if medical personnel perceive the illness differently from the patient or the family" (p. 30).

A PERSPECTIVE FOR FAMILY UNDERSTANDING

Unfortunately, not all family members who are ill or disabled are "loved ones". The identified patient may be a family member whose life has been characterized by chaos and dysfunction, whose lifelong behavior prior to the onset of the illness or disability may have had a central role in causing the family distress and problems. In some cases these behaviors may have been a factor in the cause of the illness and disability as well as other familial losses and traumas. For example, the neglect of a dysfunctional mother or father may have resulted in a severe burn for a child who was left at home alone. How does one repair the mind, body, and spirit while living on a daily basis with the life-long effect of poor judgment or inappropriate behavior?

It is important to consider this perspective when attempting to access and involve the family as a resource during the treatment and rehabilitation process. This is especially so when the family realizes that ongoing involvement is a process of reliving what has occurred and experiencing more guilt and blame, and is, in effect, more of a burden than an opportunity. This point was illustrated by the following statements by persons faced with the transformation of a family member consequent to the occurrence of an illness and disability:

> You were supposed to be watching the children, and not racing a boat on the lake. It is all your fault they got into our boat and you were too cheap to buy the extra life vests. One dead and one crippled for life! How can we ever live with this?

How can I ever forgive you? You were drunk and three of our children were burned to death and the other two will spend years in surgery. It does not matter that you have stopped drinking now!

If you did not divorce me, our son would not be lying here dying. I would never have let him have a motorcycle and you did. God has punished you.

What kind of a grandmother are you? I left my only child with you and he almost drowns in the lake. Now he is very limited and my life is ruined. Are you going to care for him the rest of his life? (Note the grandmother said "yes" and has done this for 34 years.

I told you that we should have a medical plan. Now what are we suppose to do? You quit your job to find yourself and in the process you have destroyed the family and all of our futures.

A PERSPECTIVE OF FAMILY RESILIENCE

Often the key to the successful negotiation of the change and loss process is how resilient the individual and collective family members are, or can become (Power & Dell Orto, 2003). Defining family resilience in the context of change and crisis, McCubbin and McCubbin (1988) stated: "Characteristics, dimensions, and properties of families which help families to be resistant to disruption in the face of change and adaptive in the face of crisis situations" (p. 27). Hawley and Dehann (1996) presented resilience in a developmental context:

Family resilience describes the path a family follows as it adapts and prospers in the face of stress, both in the present and over time. Resilient families respond positively to these conditions in unique ways, depending on the context, developmental level, the interactive combination of risk and protective factors, and the family, shared outlook (p. 293).

Hawley and Dehann (1996) also emphasized the importance of context in understanding how families will respond to stressful events: "Therefore it is impossible to make assumptions or predictions based on the knowledge of certain events, without understanding how that event interacts with other life circumstances" (p. 289).

A PERSPECTIVE OF AFFIRMATION

Thematic to the context of the following chapters, it is the authors' belief that for some families the experience of illness and disability can be reconceptualized and not considered just as a tragedy, but also as an opportunity to transcend the constraints of their situation and roles. The illness/disability event can be viewed as a shared experience and understanding of barriers, a time when individual family members can determine lifestyles, make affirmative choices, and develop expectations that can take control of support and related service resources (Swain & French, 2000). In order to better understand and cope with the complexities related to intense and pervasive losses, moreover, changes that are consequent to many illnesses and disabilities could be thought more as conditions of living which, in turn, will give families and society a chance to validate humanity and to cope gracefully and with dignity. Illness and disability have the potential to challenge familial belief systems because of their complexity, intensity, irrationality, and often long-term nature. These characteristics force families to make major structured adjustments to accommodate the emerging needs of the family member who has experienced the illness and disability and must live with its life altering effects.

Taylor, Kemeny, Reed, Bower, and Gruenewald (2000) stated:

> Most of the research that has related psychosocial factors to changes in disease states has focused on negative psychological states, including depression, stress, grief, and loneliness. Yet, philosophers and increasingly scientists as well have noted that exposure to trauma and other stressful life events do not inevitably lead to depression and despair. Such experiences can also act as catalysts for revaluation of one's goals and priorities and for reestablishing a sense of self. . . . Increasing evidence indicates that the array of positive outcomes that may result from stressful events include finding meaning in life, developing better coping skills, enhancing one's social resources, establishing priorities, and recognizing the value of social relationships" (p. 106).

It is important to note, however, that existing service delivery systems and programs cannot meet all the needs of all families all of the time, and it is unreasonable to expect that they do so. What is not unreasonable is that families should have options, as well as opportunities to access those resources that can minimize the unnecessary frustrations, disappointments, and heartache, and facilitate the conditions of stabilization, acceptance, growth, survival, resilience, and recovery. In some situations the advantage of a personal trauma is that it can create a vision based on hope and dreams, not just resignation. Rolland (1994) makes this point when he reflected on his medical training:

> I did not really learn to appreciate the many dilemmas and strains for families with serious health problems until my personal life was directly affected.

Within one year my mother had a stroke and my first wife was diagnosed with an incurable form of cancer. I was totally unprepared for the strains of coping with my family member's life-threatening illnesses (p. xii).

CONCLUSION

To better understand and cope with the complexities related to intense and pervasive losses, the changes and opportunities consequent to many illnesses and disabilities must be viewed as conditions of living. Such perspectives will give families an opportunity to operationalize their potential for resilience and assist family members in making the transition from loss to opportunity, from desperation to hope, and from frustration to acceptance. For a family living with the illness and disability experience, moreover, the treatment and rehabilitation process is a sequence of demands, unknowns, challenges, disappointments, as well as rewards. Fortunately there has been an increase in the realization that the family has a vital role in negotiating this process and experience.

It is one of the main tenets of this book that it is a challenge to help families negotiate the periods of life, living, and loss without losing an affirmative perspective, purpose, sense of self, and soul. No burden is too great that it cannot be redefined and renegotiated. The goal is to have a meaningful destination and not be forced to make the journey alone. While the sudden onset of an anticipated or unanticipated illness or disability cannot be undone, nor can irrational causes such as violence be completely eradiated, the support needed by families to cope with an illness or disability certainly can and must be improved. The key question to ask is where, when, and how families are going to find the support, role models, resources, encouragement, and skills needed to confront and manage the emotional and physical perils of the health care and rehabilitation process. Fortunately, there has been the emergence of new ports in this storm that certainly make the process more reasonable, bearable, and survivable (Weihs, Fisher, & Baird 2002). Added to this emergence is a philosophy of assisting families in illness and disability situations that emphasizes an affirmation of the experience and a search for new opportunities. In 2003, many problems related to living with illness and disabilities have been solved, other have been created, and some are yet to emerge. As members of the health and human care professions, and as partners with the people and the families we work with and serve, it is necessary to understand, as well as appreciate the enormous challenge related to coping with illness and disability within a familial as well as a life and living context.

JANET: DEALING WITH SPINA BIFIDA

MAINTAINING A BALANCED ATTITUDE

Maintaining a balanced attitude as a family member while experiencing the continued impact of a chronic illness or severe disability is crucial to effective coping. Achieving this balanced outlook while confronting the many realities associated with a serious medical condition is an endless struggle. In this chapter these realities have been conceptualized as perspectives, such as vulnerability, family challenges, stress, family change, and relationships with health care professionals. In turn, these realities also become a foundation for family understanding, resilience, and affirmation. The mother's story in the following account identifies the many perspectives highlighted in the chapter, and illustrates how the awareness of changes, stressors, and one's vulnerability can stimulate understanding and resilience.

*****

Both my husband and I have come from upper-middle class families of four children; he is the youngest of four boys, and I am the oldest child in my family. Each of us has also compensated for a mild form of disability. Although I remember almost no direct conversations regarding my congenital hearing loss, I was taken regularly to Boston for tests and treatments. Probably before my school years I had taught myself to read lips and to stay close to people whose words I wanted to hear. Reading difficulties plagued my husband during his school years, and he received tutoring and summer help. He, too, was able to succeed in school, intellectually able to fine-tune his auditory learning abilities. We each made a practice of "passing" as normal, choosing instead to work around the difficulties.

At the time of our marriage I was 21^1/$_2$ years old and my fiancé was 29. Our courtship had been a relatively short ten months. Although we attempted to expand our family shortly after marriage, there were problems. Pregnancy difficulties over 6 years were the first problems that either of us had really come across that could not be resolved by working harder. Action oriented, we tried all medical possibilities from tests to surgeries, capitalizing on the hope of each. We became closer than most couples, I think, but the closeness was largely nonverbal, as we rarely discussed our disappointments but could see it in each others' faces, especially during the many times in the hospital, sitting quietly, sometimes holding hands. We considered it a sign of strength that we could maintain our optimistic façade, especially with others, even members of our families of origin who visited but were not overly attentive.

The most difficult trial during our early marriage occurred when I had to have emergency surgery for a ruptured ectopic pregnancy that could have ended my life. I was more concerned that the surgery ended not only the pregnancy but also our chances for having children at all. Aware only of a sense of defeat and questions about what to do with my life, I sought no further than my husband and the doctor for support for my bruised self-esteem. Initiating adoption procedures and keeping busy did help to fend off some of the discouragement.

The following fall another pregnancy began against all medical odds. This pregnancy, like the others, got off to a troublesome start, and we didn't dare hope it would continue. It did continue, however, even without any medical intervention, for which we would later be glad. As each month passed, and we could feel the baby moving, we became more and more sure that our troubles were over. By seven months we felt as if we were home free, because even babies born that early often survived unscathed. We went through Lamaze classes together. Those months in the last half of the pregnancy will probably always be remembered as our happiest, closest, and most deliciously carefree with both of us wrapped up in the event to come. Beth's delivery was "medically unremarkable." For us it was a most remarkable achievement, all the more worthy because we had warded off all anesthesia and even the threatened forceps. Yet even as we congratulated each other and snapped a photo or two in the delivery room, we registered the silence of the staff that came only moments before the doctor told us what he had just discovered: Beth had been born with a meningomyelocele (open spine).

The obstetrician was kind and gentle, putting his hand on my arm as he told us of the meningomyelocele. He told us nothing more, and my strong biology background registered a thud in the back of my mind but did not connect. All I could ask was whether Beth would be all right, whether she would live, to which I received affirmative answers. On a maternal high, I found the nurses to be annoyingly businesslike and was glad to finally return to my room to make phone calls. My husband was back with me when we were told the baby would be sent by ambulance to Boston, and even then we assumed that Beth would be hospitalized for whatever was necessary and would come home later fine. The pediatrician arrived and began the jumble of what was to be our introduction to spina bifida. Although I recall that he gave a long description of the many organs and functions affected by the condition,

I remember little else except his kindness and brutal honesty. A voice in my head kept repeating, "My baby won't be like that," and I was worrying about my husband, who had also been up all night and was expected to accompany the baby to Boston.

My husband will never forget that trip to Boston, being asked whether to treat the baby- a decision, really, whether to let her live. He was told she was paralyzed from the waist down, would never walk, and would be retarded if she lived at all- and then he had to return to me to go through it all again. With essentially no guidance from anyone, we were asked to make a decision regarding a child for whom we had waited for six years and about a condition we had never heard of until just hours earlier. Coming to an agreement was only the first of many extreme difficulties, as we juggled our high value on this child against a future we could not begin to imagine. Beth's back was closed at the age of 24 hours. With this commitment I resolved that if she were to be disabled, at least I would see to it that she maximized every potential.

In those early days we did not cope; we existed. Minute followed minute and crisis followed crisis. We tried to keep up with our social life in an effort to maintain some semblance of an old reality, but I found those times dreamlike and irrelevant, because I was unable to think of anything but Beth and us. My husband appeared to me to be intensely emotional, but he kept it in tight control; it was too big for us to discuss in anything but small snatches.

Our families were in their own shock and did not know how to help. Nor did we know how to ask for help. Our mothers visited Beth and me in the hospital, and I was grateful, especially sensing that they were ill equipped to deal with the horror stories of others packed in around us at the nursery. I at least had had a medical background and could better understand both the hope and the limits of care given in answer to the insistent beeping of monitors. Meanwhile, our siblings received contradictory misinformation and tended either to minimize or exaggerate the facts of Beth's condition. Many people, family included, came to us with success stories about other children with spina bifida. Although I acknowledged their intent to help with hope, I also made a very conscious effort to put out of my mind these other stories, knowing that Beth was an individual and would be in her own way different from any others.

Within days of Beth's birth, our entire value system changed abruptly. All issues, problems, questions were related to matters of life and death. Nothing seemed more important than survival. Concurrently, the value we placed on friendship skyrocketed, as there seemed so few people who could even begin to understand what we were going through. I seemed to live at a layer many levels deeper and more vulnerable than ever before and became acutely sensitive, while at the same time attempting an incongruous façade of strength. We learned quickly that others needed to be put at ease with us, because they felt inadequate to help. Most did not know whether to send us a baby gift or flowers for condolence, whereas what was really important was that they cared enough to send anything. As time went on, I found, and still find, more and more people with problems of many kinds turning to me for solace, because they know somehow that I have grown sensitive ears.

In her first 18 months, Beth had nine operations, including brain surgery for a shunt and two revisions for the hydrocephalus that developed at three weeks. She seemed to spend more time in the hospital than out of it. Two or three times when she had severe urinary tract infections, I opted to keep her at home and give her injections around the clock to avoid another hospitalization. Carrying out a relentless litany of medical procedures, equipment applications, exercises, treatments, and medication administrations, I have never ceased to be amazed at what one can learn to consider an ordinary part of life. Part of what was most difficult was keeping track of the constant changes. When she first came home at the age of six weeks, I initially had little confidence in caring for this small girl. It felt as if she belonged more to the hospital than to us. The staff had been very supportive in teaching me, though, and by the end of the first year I had gained some considerable expertise. My life was lived more moment-to-moment than day to day, with a motto of, "Tomorrow may not be any better, but at least it'll be different," or, "At least I'll never be bored." Planning even a day in advance was difficult because there were so many appointments and changes. But by the end of the first year I had developed a technique I called "putting my worries on hold." I was able to make an observation of impending crisis, set a reasonable time for a new evaluation of the problem, and mentally put aside anxiety on the issue until the appointed time and the new information. I would then (1) act, (2) decide it was a false alarm, or (3) go back on hold until the next assessment. I was determined to "accept" her condition and to avoid foisting my hang-ups on her, and to the extent that even at my worst I have managed to keep her independence in sight as my first priority for her, I have been fairly successful in maintaining an attitude of optimism and open honesty. Emotionally speaking, however, the first year was relatively easy, with numbness and denial carrying me along.

My husband, meanwhile, pulled together after the initial weeks into a stable strength. His attitude is generally more pessimistic and fatalistic than my complementary optimist activism. To this day, he starts with the worst possibilities and works toward reality, whereas I look to the most hopeful, backtracking toward reality where we meet minds. Although I do not entirely understand his ability to mentally analyze a problem and work toward a solution alone, I do see that this method works for him. Says he about problems, "I think about them alone, in the car, uninterrupted, and I break the cycle" of going round and round on the same issue. On the other hand, he does not entirely understand my need to, as he puts it, "Sit around and talk about the same things."

When Beth was 18 months old, she had to have double hip surgery, necessitating use of a spica cast and a Bradford frame for two months. Concurrently, my husband was laid up with what was later diagnosed as a broken back, which could have left him a paraplegic as well. Both were in body casts at the same time. It was then that I began to seriously doubt my ability to continue. We had also just begun Beth's program of intermittent catheterization primarily to avoid what we considered to be destructive surgery on her bladder. Although I became tied to the schedule and even the urologist was skeptical, Beth had far fewer infections. More tired than I ever knew was possible, I also felt especially lonely with my husband seeming to be someone else when he was on high doses of painkillers. My life seemed to consist of nothing besides constant nursing duties, and I knew that I was not functioning at all well.

Until this time I had had very little in the way of external support besides medical expertise and a few select baby-sitters on whom I depended heavily for some time out. My husband and I have insisted on maintaining some semblance of a social life, with some time set aside for just the two of us. We have both found it essential to our sanity and to our marriage in spite of financial pressures and hassles in getting sitters. We have had extraordinarily good luck with training students in high school or college. I hide nothing from them and describe what is involved to check their reactions before actually teaching them and putting them to work. For privacy's sake we have insisted on having only girls involved with the catheterization and find that once they have matured a bit beyond their own self-consciousness over puberty, they accept our medical regime matter-of-factly.

Through our Lamaze teacher I became involved with an organization of parents of special-needs children. I had, of course, met many other parents of disabled children and had had meaningful conversations at clinics, in hospital corridors, and occasionally on the phone, but there was no sense of continuity with these people who were not otherwise parts of our lives. After a lecture sponsored by Parent to Parent on the subject of birth defects, I discovered a sense of warm, interested, understanding community spirit among the local parents in over an

hour of conversation. The parents were as varied as the special needs
their children represented. It was exhilarating to be face-to-face with a
group of sane people who could cope (something I very much needed
to know how to do), people who were just as much in awe of my situation
as I was of theirs. Parent to Parent also helped open many doors to
worlds of assorted resources. Even though I had since the beginning
specialized in becoming an expert on the subjects of spina bifida and
hydrocephalus from a medical standpoint, through the parent group
I began to learn of consumer services, sources of adaptive equipment
and clothing, and helpful hints to facilitate the translation of medical
treatment into individual family living.

By the time Beth was two and a half, our lives had stabilized some-
with my husband back on his feet and Beth home for a whole year
without hospitalization. I went to an exercise class and became satisfy-
ingly involved with Parent to Parent, matching families for phone support. With assistance through an Early Intervention program Beth had
begun to walk with a walker and braces to the waist, and her developmental age was gaining on her chronological age. During this time, we
got a call from the adoption agency telling us that they had a three
week old baby girl for us to pick up in just four days. She was adorable
and very much wanted, even so suddenly, but those first months were
awfully hectic for me, because Lindsey had her own set of problems;
colic from the start, pneumonia requiring hospitalization at the age of
ten weeks, four months of incessant crying, and finally the discovery of
her allergy to milk that lasted until she was over two years old. Actually,
now I am glad for these problems because they established immediately
a place for Lindsey in our family, which might otherwise have tended
to put aside her needs for Beth's, which still seemed so urgent. Always,
even during the hardest times, I knew that Lindsey's assertive presence
was beneficial to all of us, although I worried about whether she got
enough attention. I felt somewhat saddened and slightly cheated that
Lindsey and I would never be as intimately involved as Beth and I had
been. It was my husband who helped me see that I was over-involved
with Beth, not that Lindsey was lacking my attention. Both girls were
thriving, Beth as the oldest, Lindsey with the attentions of a big sister.

Once I gained some time and the distance that Beth's schooling
provided at age three and a half, I was able to see our enmeshment
more clearly. I had not been prepared for the sense of responsibility
I would feel toward a child, perhaps even an able-bodied one. The
enmeshment had been understandably born out of our desires for a
child and the related needs of this particular one. Enmeshment was
also fostered by the system that taught me all the care and treatments.

I once realized that I was expected to carry out nine hours of assorted treatments per day, while meals, baths, groceries, a social life, laundry, errands and recreation were to come out of the little remaining time. The diluting effect of Lindsey's arrival had been very healthy. My husband's role and mine did not change a great deal, but they expanded instead to include more tasks, some of which were traded or shared. He spent many hours each week on the paper work and financial mix-ups of insurance, handicapped license plates, taxes, and the like.

By the time Beth was five and Lindsey two and a half, I was mired in depression. My previously optimistic ability to make the most of a hard situation had burned out in negative musings on how badly we would lose this game of life with a disabled child in spite of all the hard work. To my credit, I knew even then that Beth's disability was far from the whole problem (scapegoating), but I also knew that I needed professional help. I had read many times about the grief surrounding the birth of a child with defects, but the literature did not ring true for me. My life certainly included denial, anger, bargaining, depression, and acceptance. But for me these were not milestones on a timeline, but were aspects of every day, sometimes every hour. Furthermore, there was little grief attached to the "expected baby." The grief was tied up in the whole mental picture I had had for my family, our future, and myself. Feeling I had failed myself, my husband, Beth, the family, and even society itself, what I really had lost was my whole sense of self-worth, which I defined in terms of what I could do.

The most significant help came to me through a fine clinical psychologist who worked individually with me, primarily on the issue of self-esteem, helping me to better integrate my thinking with my feelings. From the start he offered me respect, as if I had as much to teach him as he had to teach me, and he responded with compassion and human reactions, from time to time with tears in his eyes. His positive regard for me supported his assumption that I could grow through this, and that, indeed, I already had. I was certain that I had crossed the line into insanity, wishing I could quietly evaporate. He got me an antidepressant, which helped me to go on and see that all of the overwhelming things I was feeling were, even in all their intensity, normal reactions to abnormal circumstances. The counselor taught me a whole new perspective on worth and value, one that rested on who I am, not on what I do. From this viewpoint then, failures or disapproval could not change my value as a person.

Crucial to the counseling was my somewhat private but strong faith in God, a faith shared by the counselor but not by my husband. Rigidly clinging to various misconceptions, I was less able to utilize effectively the resources of my faith. For instance, guilt was not an issue for me intellectually or even spiritually, because I believe in forgiveness. But emotionally I felt I deserved this disaster, not realizing I also had to forgive myself. I learned about peace and pacing as well as about my own human limitations, and I relearned a sense I had had long ago, that there is something to be learned in every situation. Knowing I was doing the best I could under the circumstances, I could let God take over the responsibility for the end results and put aside long-term worries. The counselor helped me gain a perspective, a broader sense of time and meaning for my life. Contemplating the biblical concept of unconditional love also helped bolster my sense of self-esteem. By the time we terminated, I was able to see myself as a special and unique individual, equipped with my own set of strengths and weaknesses, grown and growing. These gifts could actually be used for the benefit of others, and a future began to form for the first time in five years. I had never before seen myself in this light, and it was a monumental turning point for me. Also, a growing involvement with our local church provided not just spiritual sustenance, but practical assistance and a warm, new support network as well.

The interaction between the girls has been decidedly normal, although frequently they seem closer than do many sisters, sharing well and at times showing surprising consideration for each other. Beth's time in school has given me a chance to be with just Lindsey and to delight in her development, which, although less studied than Beth's, has been remarkable in its own right. The two of them fight and squabble like any other siblings and also gang up against us parents. It is a loud, irritating nuisance, but I realize a sense of gratefulness that they can be so normal. That each has an effect on the other is clear. In a burst of independence and perhaps competition with her sister, Beth learned to catheterize herself last fall, but tries on occasion to go "like Lindsey" without a catheter. Lindsey in the meantime was very slow in toilet training, and I wondered if she craved the attention Beth got at the toilet. Although I have made a concerted effort to help each view herself as an individual, I am seldom sure of how life looks from their angle.

I have also tried to direct disability-related anger at the equipment or the spina bifida itself, as opposed to Beth herself. I don't know yet whether she can herself make the distinction. She said several months ago, "I hate meatballs, applesauce, and myself," then paused while my ears pricked up and added, "I don't know why I said that, Mummy." As casually as I could, I asked her what she didn't like about herself. "Oh." she thought, "casts and braces and catheters and stuff." We talked it out, cried it out, as I tried to help her separate these things from whom she is. A few weeks later she asked, "Mummy, how come you always like to talk to me about braces and crutches and spina bifida?" Perception is perhaps Beth's greatest strength, and I knew as I chuckled that I'd been had. Yet it wasn't much later that she said, "You know, Mum, there are some good things about spina bifida. I get lots and lots of extra attention."

In the meantime, Lindsey is becoming quite the athlete, and I have wondered how Beth would take to her sister's prowess on bikes, skis and roller skates. Beth has opted to try each to the best of her ability with our help, and since Lindsey's first steps "without anything," Beth has so far been quite proud of her sister. In a thousand little ways, such as grocery shopping (Who rides in the cart? Who walks?), my husband and I have also had to face Lindsey's passing Beth in abilities, and we are reminded that it is personhood that is important, not abilities. With this in mind, I can freely encourage Lindsey's weekly swimming with more enthusiasm that I might otherwise have.

My husband and I, like Beth and Lindsey, lead parts of our lives together and other parts more separately. We have mustered a fairly united front in house rules and discipline. Now that I am out of the house more, having returned to school with the goal of eventually re-joining the work force, my husband has to pick up more of the childcare and household chores. Conversely, I hope in time to provide some income to offset the pressures on him. Although it is still difficult to predict the future for either of our children, we have a hopeful coincid-ing picture of independence for each. We may be wrong, but we have probably considered a full spectrum of possible outcomes, although we don't look too far ahead. The more I study, the more I come to the comforting conviction that, despite some asynchrony, our family is in-deed generally functional. It is far from perfect, and nothing is ever that simple. However, a strong alliance in our marriage, our flexibility, and the healthy dyads in each direction can all help build our coping strengths. These years, although frequently overwhelming, have been a challenge to growth for each of us. Frankly, I am proud of the maturity we have each gained. I become more and more convinced that the lessons most worth learning are also the most painful ones. The pain will undoubtedly continue, but so, too, I think, will the growth.

DISCUSSION QUESTIONS

1. What were the factors that you believe contributed to the parents' vulnerability? Do you feel they experienced a "sense" of vulnerability?

2. Were the sources of stress more from the nature of the child's disability than from the personality of the mother or father, or the lack of care giving experience?
3. When did the mother change and have more of a balanced perspective towards caring for her daughter?
4. What factors contributed to this family's resilience?

Imagine that you are a health professional who is going to meet with the mother and father described in this Personal Statement in the hospital after their child experienced a severe urinary tract infection which is being successfully treated. The parents are very disappointed and appear emotionally drained. When speaking with them, what would you wish to emphasize?

SET 1: CURING ILLNESS AND DISABILITY

PERSPECTIVE

What if an experimental treatment was discovered that could eliminate the effects of spina bifida as well as some other illnesses or disabilities. The cost is $200,000 per year. Would such an experiment have made a difference in their family life with their child?

EXPLORATION

1. Who should pay for the treatment?
2. How should people be selected for treatment?
3. Should severity of the condition be considered?
4. If a person had multiple disabilities such as spina bifida, mental retardation, and severe mental illness should they be given priority or be excluded?
5. Should a hospital or rehabilitation facility be limited in the amount of money it could charge for this treatment?

REFERENCES

Baider, L., Kaufman, B., Peretz, T., Manor, O., Ever-Hadani, P., & Kaplan-DeNour,
(1996). Mutuality of fate: Adaptation and psychological distress in cancer patients

and their partners: In L. Baider, C. Cooper, & A. Kaplan-DeNour (Eds.). *Cancer and the family*, (pp 173-186). Chichester, England: John Wiley & Sons, Ltd.

Boss, P., Caron, W., Horbal, J., & Mortimer, J. (19990). Predictors of depression in caregivers of dementia patients: Boundary ambiguity and master. *Family Process*, 29 (3), 245-254.

Connell, G. M., & Connell, L. C. (1995). In hospital consultation: Systemic intervention during medical crisis, *Family Systems Medicine*, *13*(1), 29–32

Garwick, A. W., Patterson, J., Bennet, F. C., & Blum, R. W. (1995). Breaking the news: How families first learn about their child's chronic condition. *Archives of Pediatric & Adolescent Medicine*, *149*(9), 991–997.

Hawley, D. R., & Dehann, L. (1996). Toward a definition of family resilience: Integrating life - span and family perspectives. *Family Process*, *35*(3), 283–298.

Helgeson, V.S. (1994). The onset of chronic illness: Its effect on the patient-spouse relationship. *Journal of Social and Clinical Psychology*, 12 (4), 406-428.

McCubbin, H., & McCubbin, M. (1988). Typologies of resilient families: Emerging roles for social class and ethnicity. *Family Relations*, *37*, 247–254.

McDaniel, S. H., Hepworth, J., & Doherty, W. J. (1999). The shared emotional themes of illness, *Journal of Family Psychotherapy*, *10*(4), 1–8.

Power, P. W., & Dell Orto, A. E. (2003). *The resilient family: Living with your child's illness or disability*. Notre Dame, IN: Sorin Press.

Rocchio, C. (1998) Can families manage behavioral programs in home settings, *Brain Injury Source*, *2*(4), 34–35.

Rolland, J. S. (1994) *Families, illness and disability*. New York: Basic Books.

Swain, J., & French, S. (2000). Toward an affirmation model of disability. *Journal of Disability and Society*, *15*(4), 569–582.

Taylor, S. E., Kemeny, M. E., Reed, G. M., Bower, J. E., & Gruenewald, T. L. (2000). Psychological resources, positive illusions and health. *American Psychologist*, *55*(1), 99–121.

Weihs, K., Fisher, L., & Baird, M. (2002). Families health, and behavior: A section of the commissioned report by the Committee on Health and Behavior: Research, Practice, and Policy. *Families, Systems & Health*, *20*(1), 7–46.

Zemzars, I. S. (1984). Adjustment to health loss: Implications for psychosocial treatment. In S. E. Milligan (Ed.), *Community health care for chronic physical illness: Issues and models*, Cleveland, OH: Case Western Reserve University.

2

Children With Disabilities
and the Family

Today more than 20 million children and adolescents are living with a chronic illness or severe disability. The large number of illnesses varies in prevalence from being extremely rare to quite common (Gaither, Bingan, & Hopkins, 2000). Because of medical advances, most of these young people will live into adulthood. Though children and adolescents who experience severe illness and disability related traumas have a unique array of adaptive patterns, it is the family who usually must bear the primary care-giving responsibilities. The family is the most important source of support and developmental impetus (Lustig, 2002). The family is also instrumental in achieving a balance between the illness/disability related demands and all the members' quality of life. On the other hand, the daily tasks associated with maintaining this balance can seriously affect the marital relationship and overall productive, family functioning. A complex situation is often created for family members, and parents especially are at great risk of experiencing marital distress (Cloutier, Manion, Walker, & Johnson, 2002). In turn, lack of support and cohesion within the family, parental psychopathology, and couple conflict have been identified as stressors for children (Gaither, Bingen, & Hopkins, 2000).

In the ideal world or in our hopes and expectations, children and adolescents are not supposed to be ill, disabled, or at risk. They are expected to be healthy, reasonably happy, and embody the joys and energy of life. Unfortunately, this is not always the case and this population is a significant part of the health care system. This chapter will discuss two key realities when confronting illness/disability and the health care system: the child/adolescent and their available family. A specific focus will be on the range of emotions, stressors, and needs that young people and other family members experience when dealing both with the medical condition itself and its collateral damage. An understanding of these behaviors and constructs (stressors and needs) provides a perspective for identifying the family's adaptive processes. In turn, these processes suggest guidelines for effective interventions directed to appropriate adjustment for all family members.

DETERMINANTS AND INFLUENCES ON CHILD/ADOLESCENT REACTION AND FAMILY ADAPTIVE PROCESSES TO ILLNESS AND DISABILITY

Both determinants of and influences on the emotional reaction to a chronic illness or disability should be viewed in a developmental perspective. The impact of an illness or disability can be more or less problematic depending on the stage of development of the child and the effect on the developmental tasks. Younger children may be more vulnerable to severe effects from major illness and traumas than adolescents because they may have less fully developed life skills. Because of these developmental differences, understanding the emergence of individual reactions is complex. There are certain determinants that represent themes found in pre-injury and injury characteristics of young people which can provide guidelines to understanding illness and disability related behaviors and concerns, with the exception of age and developmental issues. For children and adolescents with congenital conditions, the influences are generally the same as for those with acquired severe medical conditions (Lustig, 2002).

NATURE AND SEVERITY OF INJURY

The degree of physical impairment, whether the medical condition is life threatening or has a predicted or uncertain course of the disability, will affect the young person and the family's reaction. Significant changes to motor-sensory skills, intellectual and physical functioning, and communication abilities may result in very frustrating situations which are further compounded by a lack of motivation to undertake many life tasks. Difficulties in controlling the management of the chronic illness add stress both to the young person and other family members. The physical aspect of the medical condition may be particularly important for adolescents who are very concerned with body image. As a young man with facial scarring from severe burns said, "I was so despondent over how others were seeing me that I wanted to kill myself. But fortunately I had some role models who helped me appreciate that life could be worth living" (Breakey, 1997).

AGE AND DEVELOPMENTAL ISSUES

The concept of age includes the emotional adjustment of the young person at the onset of the medical condition. Age can determine how children or adolescents confront returning to school following a trauma and how they engage in complex and advanced learning challenges. There are certain developmental tasks associated with age groups, and how one has learned these tasks prior to an injury can make a difference in post-injury adjustment. Also, secure children who believe they are understood and accepted by their parents may adapt more easily to the limitations imposed by the disability or chronic illness than young people who have conflicted feelings or perceive a clear sense of rejection regarding parental acceptance. Experiences in the family circle strongly affect a young person's competence and self-esteem.

A developmental trend influencing the young person's response to a severe disability of illness is the individual's ability to self-manage the medical and socio-emotional aspects of the condition (Miller, 1995). Active participation will help these young people to develop a sense of effectiveness and control of their bodies, to the degree possible, contributing to healthy physical and psychosocial development. Such participation will vary, of course, depending on the age and capability of the child. Preschool, elementary school, and adolescent young people have different capacities to acquire the necessary information to manage the illness and the confidence to assert themselves (Miller, 1995). Yet involvement in their treatment regimen can affect their self-esteem and even identity.

In adolescence the move toward independence becomes a powerful driving force. While there are issues of separation/alienation, body image, sexual identity, aggression, and educational and vocational development, the presence of a severe disability or chronic illness may aggravate these potential problems. Feelings of disempowerment, threat, and vulnerability are caused when assistance with many activities of daily living is needed. For an adolescent who is coping with the effects of a disability and who may be less self-assured, there is additional difficulty in resolving questions emerging from maintaining self-esteem. There are also the daily challenges of satisfying the need for companionship and peer support, and this satisfaction may often become frustrating or even unrealistic.

PSYCHOSOCIAL ENVIRONMENT

The family environment, friends, peers, the school, and health care providers represent influences that can promote manageable reactions to the young person's severe disability or illness, or a sustained, negative response leading to a long period of maladaptive patterns (Patterson & Garwick, 1998). Though each "resource" of the environment has its own distinctive contribution to the young person's emotional response and eventual adjustment (Miller, 1995), thematic to each one are attitudes and expectations from family members, friends, teachers, school administrators, and health care professionals. Negative attitudes engendered by fear, stigma, and stereotyping may have a devastating effect on how the young person handles self-care and his or her self-esteem Positive attitudes and expectations contribute to acceptance and a sense of worth. But each resource provides a particular influence on the young person's response to the serious medical condition.

The Family Environment

The family is the most important source of support and a powerful companion to health providers and the school in assisting the child/adolescent to respond in an adaptive way (Gaither, Bingen, & Hopkins, 2000; Miller, 1995). But many young people do not have fully functioning families who are capable of meeting the everyday demands of care giving. The role of significant others may have to fill this void. The family's adjustment, however, can be a primary determinant for the emotional adjustment of the child or adolescent. Family instability, parents' psychiatric history, socioeconomic status, and child-rearing practices all contribute to post-injury quality of life. Parents who have available support resources, stability, and education may minimize the at-risk quality of problematic adjustment patterns. The parents' emotional resources can be drained by care giving demands, leaving little time for the adjustment demands of their other children. Parents who have a developed ability for tolerance and empathy and who understand the effects of a disability and the distinctive needs of their other children contribute to a home environment that is more conducive to the care giving demands of the child or adolescent.

Children or adolescents with a disability or chronic illness and with parents who are separated, divorced, or remarried, though a common experience in today's society, may have distinctive needs. The questions of who has primary care giving responsibilities and the problems concerned with how conflicts caused by marital discord can be minimized should be addressed for the purposes of the young person's welfare. Conflicts between divorced parents or everyday problems that may be caused by joint custody can have a negative impact on the child and chronic illness adjustment concerns. These concerns can be further complicated when a child becomes severely injured while in the custody of one parent.

There are also family, ethnic, and cultural influences that may have a positive or negative effect on the young person's quality of life (Harry, 2002). For example, particular cultural groups place an important emphasis on the extended family's availability in times of loss or serious injury. The extended family acts as a buffer that modulates those stressful periods in home life that, in turn, contributes to the young person's quality of life. On the other hand, because of culturally based beliefs, if the family perceives illness and disability as a punishment or stigma, the child and family can be further stressed and isolated. It is most important that the helping professional understand the family's cultural background so that the factors that promote adaptive functioning can be identified.

Frequently lost in any discussion of family dynamics and disability is the reaction of siblings to the sister or brother's severe disability or chronic illness. This reaction may significantly affect families and can have implications for other children's functioning. Having a sibling with a disability may add to the young person's emotional distress, perceived threat, personal responsibility, and adjustment problems (Cohen, 1999; Nixon & Cummings, 1999). Birth order, gender, and family size may be predictive of the objective and subjective burden and the socioemotional adjustment of nonhandicapped siblings. Such issues as embarrassment over the behavior of the brother or sister, guilt for not being the injured one, and resentment for not receiving as much attention as the injured, are concerns that impact the family. Further distress occurs when the children become the sounding board for their parents' grief and frustration, especially when there is a single parent (Patterson, 1988). These problems cause stress within the family environment that, in turn, affect the adjustment of the young person. Other families have been enriched by the support and caring concern of siblings.

School Issues

The school environment is the center for intellectual and academic development. The way in which the school responds to the child or adolescent's disability or chronic illness will affect quality of life and medical management (Miller, 1995). Entry or re-entry into the school system can be a very significant hurdle to overcome (Clarke, 1996). Problems with academic achievement may not be apparent for a year or more after disability/illness onset, so when they are detected they may not be attributed to the trauma. When faced with newly acquired deficits as well as assets, survivors and their families may be forced to change their expectations of themselves. With the growing number of young people with disabilities entering the education system, challenges emerge regarding the educator's knowledge as to how a disability can affect a student's academic and social functioning. Appropriate information to the educator about the young person's medical condition can make a difference in this individual's overall adjustment. Establishing communication links between the family, health professionals, and the school is an important step to helping the child/adolescent manage the medical condition. Again, self-management contributes to the building of self-esteem.

Friends and Peers

Depending on the severity and complexity of the severe disability or illness, family members may overly protect a young person or peers may be overly fascinated by the illness. Such protection and fascination could also express special attention. But when the young person is confronted with the normal social interaction accompanying school and leisure activities, feelings of rejection may be created. There may also be the difficulty of "fitting in" and being accepted (Cohen, 1999).

Those who have been disabled or chronically ill since birth may have learned in their very early years how to negotiate the social system with peers. Johnson (1997) believes that for those with congenital conditions, disability completely shapes their lives, and "we take constraints that no one would choose and build rich and satisfying lives with them" (p. 419). But usually the specter of stigma and other forms of prejudice are lurking in the world of the young person with a severe disability/illness. These negative attitudes generate fear among friends, and in turn, create added feelings of rejection and isolation for the child or adolescent. Self-help groups and positive role models can be critical intervention approaches to alleviate some of these difficulties.

Health Professionals

Communication styles differ among health professionals, and a hesitancy to include the young person in medical treatment plans when it is age appropriate to do so, or a reluctance to impart necessary information that can assist the child or adolescent to meet adaptive demands, can only add to existing feelings of isolation and rejection. Anxiety on the part of the young person usually accompanies an encounter with health care providers, and this reaction needs to be addressed if the child or adolescent is to become a willing partner in self-care management. Importantly, self-care management enhances feelings of self-worth. Also, informational support provided by service providers may alleviate many family concerns (Patterson, Garwick, Bennett & Blum, 1997).

All of these determinants can trigger a wide range of emotions in the child or adolescent with severe illness/disability and in other family members. During the initial family meeting these determinants should be identified, since each one can become a guide when helping the family to assist a family member to manage the demands of living with the disability. Other factors, such as pre-injury adjustment, the length of hospitalization, and threats to the emotional needs of the young person, i.e., love and affection, self-respect, achievement, independence, and acceptance, may also contribute to the shape and intensity of the emotional reaction of the child or adolescent. Yet when all of these potential influences are recognized, they also represent a bridge, or in some instances a gateway, to the young person's world and can be pivotal in effective intervention.

DOMINANT REACTIONS AND PROBLEMS WHICH EMERGE FROM CHILD/ADOLESCENT ILLNESS AND DISABILITY

As a result of chronic illness or severe disability, there are usually many behavioral and emotional changes to the individuals. A sense of loss permeates these changes. These losses may be both interactive and cumulative. The ultimate deprivation for the young person may be the loss of a normal life span and fantasies about the way life should be (Patterson, 1988). The impact of this loss may arise during the readjustment period to school demands or the frequent interaction with peers. Progressive realization that now life is different and one may no longer have the developed ability to capably perform many activities of daily living may lead to greater social isolation and psychological loss, and thus self-esteem and hope diminish (Patterson, 1988).

Young people who may be having difficulties resuming an active life and maintaining satisfactory interpersonal relations often experience depression (Cohen, 1999). Adolescents may become withdrawn and have intense feelings of disappointment, frustration, and anger and they may feel there is little satisfaction to be derived from life. Also, changes in their behavior may be due to a restricted ability to understand many daily adjustment demands, a reduced ability for planning and self-reliance, and a difficulty in accepting dependence when there is need for independence.

Other emotional reactions of the child or adolescent, depending on the age development of the young person, are anger, grief, fear, and denial. Anger is almost an expected, powerful emotion expressed by the behaviors of pouting, silence, and moodiness. Grief is also an intense emotion, frequently masked by resentment and hostility toward others. A perception of unknown but planned medical procedures, or eventual school re-entry, may cause a lingering sense of fear. Denial of any of the implications of the medical condition may take the form that divine intervention will cause a miracle to occur. But denial can have an adaptive value, as it may temporarily reduce the fear and terror of an uncertain future. Prolonged denial, however, is not going to lead to eventual adjustment since this is often dependent on whether or not the situation improves, deteriorates, or stays the same.

The emotional reactions of the young person with a disability can precipitate serious difficulties and demands for family members, health providers, and school personnel. The adolescent's developmental struggles with sexual awareness, independence-dependence conflict, and understanding of his/her own values and lifestyle as being distinct from his/her parents, can cause continued family anxiety, disruption of family patterns, and altered parent and sibling roles. Prolonged medical treatment, often accompanied by pain and suffering, can intensify the individual's conflict with separation issues, affecting the expectations of parents toward him/her. The young person's frustration and social isolation can create tension within the family environment and inhibit the family's attempts to "right itself" and re-establish a working balance among all family members.

Because of the implications for future planning for the young person with a disability, the family realizes that hopes and dreams may have to be changed or modified. Such a transition represents a loss for family members, who grieve over the reality of long-term problems and concerns. With grief comes anger, frustration, disappointment, and depression among family members.

The young person's re-entry into the family, school, and neighborhood communities often stimulates another transitional crisis in the family. Though the child's return home and successful re-entry depends upon a close relationship between family dynamics and the child's individual behavioral integrity (Patrick and Hostler, 1998), during this transition marital conflicts, inappropriate family alliances, and un-healthy coping strategies tend to emerge. Avoiding adjustment de-mands, denying the reality of the behavioral symptoms , and displacing parental frustration on other children can only add to family disruption. Moreover, during the community re-entry phase the family may still be wondering about future prognosis as well as future risks, seeking com-plete information on the young person's problems, and figuring whether there are adequate resources to manage rehabilitation needs.

All in all, there are cognitive, emotional, and behavioral demands on the family system. These are usually combined with large financial burdens. Another factor that can affect the impact of the child's illness on the family is the length of time the parents care for a child with a chronic illness (Dahlquist, Czyzewski, & Jones, 1995). A prolonged time of caring can cause a long-term stressor that may increase in intensity. These demands create a difficult time for families, especially those with young children with complicated and long-term life care needs. Understanding complex information related to an illness or disability, being uncertain about the outcome, worrying over the future of the now "less than perfect child," and accommodating lives to the caring needs of the child represent stressors that cause a large burden on the marital relationship. Parental guilt also plays a role in development of family stressors as well as in their adaptive response (Smart, 2001). With congenital disabilities, a mother or father may believe that the cause of the disability is something they did or did not do. Much blame can circulate among the family circle, causing stress in the marital relationship and spilling over to the other children. They may feel that somehow they are responsible for the disability, and at times they are (e.g., dropping a child or not putting on seat belts).

From these emotional responses and stressors emerge selected needs for the young person and family that must be identified by family members and health care providers if the child or adolescent is to achieve an appropriate level of adjustment.

CHILD/ADOLESCENT AND FAMILY NEEDS EMERGING FROM AN ILLNESS OR DISABILITY

Though family needs have been more of a focus in the literature (Miller, 1995), the needs of the child/adolescent deserve equal attention. The emergence of these needs will depend on age developmental issues, the course of a chronic illness and the management demands of a severe disability. Each period, with its phases of "ups and downs," may stimulate a different need. But certain needs can be thematic to children and adolescents as well as several life periods, such as appropriate attention and support, security, and especially for adolescents with a severe disability or chronic illness, the need to vent feelings, to receive accurate and helpful information, to learn skills to handle selected social situations and to reduce uncertainty about the course of the medical condition. The recognition of the needs for acceptance, to establish a trusting relationship with family members, and to have available resources for nurturance can all alleviate concerns about the individuals' daily adjustment.

A significant study reported on how more than 200 families with children with TBI responded to inquiries about their current needs while managing their child's care (Pieper, 1991). The highest ranked needs were:

1. To have my questions answered honestly
2. To have complete information on my child's problems related to the disability/illness
3. To have explanations from professionals given in terms that family members can understand
4. To have enough resources for my child, such as rehabilitation programs and counseling
5. To have a professional to turn to for advice or services when my child needs help
6. To have complete information on the medical care of the child's disorder

Accurate, clear information and support services appear to be central to the needs of these parents. Families also need someone at the very beginning of the treatment and rehabilitation process to give them appropriate relevant, helpful medical information, emotional support, and practical guidance. Support services could include information and referrals, supportive counseling, and training in care giving, stress reduction, and financial management. Interestingly, when parents were asked about those services which could have been requested if they were known at injury onset, the highest demands were support groups, free health maintenance organizations, financial counseling, sibling counseling, and family counseling (Pieper, 1991).

Many of these needs, of course, often go unmet, which further contribute to family tension as attempts are made to manage daily living demands. When the child or adolescent re-enters the family after a prolonged hospitalization, and family members are confronted with the reality of the disability, expectations must be modified, special education classes should be arranged, case management concerns need attention, and sibling and parental roles are altered. Other needs surface, moreover, for family members during the post-acute rehabilitation phase. They include the assurance that their family member will be safe, allaying fear of the future, information about and assistance in obtaining adequate rehabilitation or medical insurance coverage, understanding the rehabilitation process, and the realization that they are making a positive contribution to their loved one's care (Coppa, Hepburn, Strauss, & Yody, 1999).

In attempting to fulfill their unmet needs and at the same time manage the everyday demands of living with a child or adolescent with a disability, families often come to a crossroads. Family life can either deteriorate or become more rewarding as family members restore themselves to productive, satisfying living. There are a number of factors that facilitate the families' adaptive process. As stated earlier, identifying the determinants of the child's, adolescent's, and other family members' behaviors, and recognizing their responses, behaviors, and emerging needs related to the medical situation provides a focus for understanding this adjustment process. What meaning the family gives to the congenital or adventitious disability or chronic illness can make a difference in how the family adjusts to the event. If a disability or chronic illness is only viewed as a constant source of trouble for family life, and no hope is harbored to moderate the relationship between disability-related stress and maladjustment, then constant distress may exist among family members, seriously inhibiting adaptive efforts. The belief of hope and the utilization of social support are coping resources to confront the stress of a serious disability and contribute to an interpretation of what has happened in the family resulting from disability/illness occurrence. Religious beliefs and prior assumptions about life and suffering also inject meaning into a severe disability/illness experience. More action-oriented coping resources, with individual psychological strengths, such as problem-solving skills and an inner locus of control, can assist family members to manage the environmental and internal demands prompted by the medical experience. Gaither, Bingen, and Hopkins(2000) report, however, that research suggests that having a child with chronic illness "does not necessarily have a negative impact on couple functioning" (p. 349).

There are additional factors conducive to a reasonable adjustment for family members living with the experience of a child or adolescent's severe disability and chronic illness. They are:

1. Stable family situation

   Although living with a young person with a disability can be continually disruptive, open communication among family members, a sense of security among siblings, a trusting, caring relationship among spouses, and the ability to at least manage difficult situations and perhaps capitalize on successes, all contribute to a stable family life. Such stability does not minimize unexpected periods of crisis, but a crisis has a greater probability of being managed successfully by a family that is stable, cohesive, and flexible.

2. Parent-child relationship is predominately positive

   The characteristics of this relationship include a "basic trust" established in the child, and sensitivity to the young person's needs. With frequent episodes of unpleasant or disruptive behavior, it may be very difficult to nurture this trust, but the nurturing flows from convictions that "we" want what is best for our child. An awareness of the child's or adolescent's current and emerging needs is important in building a working relationship between parent and child.

3. Parents and professionals are working cooperatively, and not at cross-purposes

   This factor presumes good communication between the professional and family members, a communication that includes realistic and helpful information available to the young person and family about the nature of the illness or disability, accessible medical, educational, and financial resources, and a clear response to questions. Parents report continued difficulties with professionals over communication issues, and health providers need to be aware of parental information needs and the ability of parents to interpret information.

4. Adequate opportunities for the young person to have peer contact and other socialization opportunities

   Parents may tend to neglect or overemphasize this aspect of the child's rehabilitation. Normalizing life patterns should be established as much as possible. This is an area that can be addressed by peer support and self-help groups.

5. The utilization of support systems, including the practice of networking

   Because of the sudden, unexpected onset of illness or disability, family members are usually not aware of available resources and how to access them. Often families are just trying to survive. Available support systems can include extended family, friends,

school or community service representatives, clergy, and networking with other family survivors. This contact helps to reduce
feelings of isolation, self-pity, and the perception that "no one
else can understand". Fears, anger, hopes, dreams, and even
unacceptable thoughts are often easier to disclose to people who
have experienced similar circumstances. To make this happen
requires a systematic outreach program that anticipates needs
rather than reacting to crisis.

6. Educational planning during the early stage of re-entry into the
    family
    Such planning can be extremely important for the young per-
    son's morale and the family's direction. Return to school is a
    major transition for the young person, but careful planning may
    minimize some of the family's anxiety over this adjustment. This
    factor assumes that school officials will be contacted as soon as
    possible after the young person's medical condition has begun
    to stabilize.

7. A realistic acceptance by the health care team of its own role,
    expectations, and needs in working with the young person and
    family members
    The health professional has an unusual impact on family mem-
    bers, for they see in this individual a source of hope and an
    anchor during the troubling adjustment family periods. Service
    providers must understand how they should respond to the varied
    family needs, and in what way they can contribute to the medical,
    educational, and many daily family concerns. For example, help-
    ing professionals can assist the family by educating and providing
    ongoing consultation to school personnel. Establishing a social
    support system for the young person can facilitate successful
    academic re-entry. Family members, however, may need help in
    learning how to confront teacher insensitivity regarding handling
    the complexities of homework with a child who has severe disabil-
    ity or chronic illness. Many school problems can be anticipated
    and prevented through scheduling modifications and appro-
    priate programming. Consequently, most families need some
    assistance in negotiating the educational system.

There is no way to consistently predict eventual "good" or "bad"
adjustment because it is a process and not a singular event. But the
family should be given the opportunity to maximize all of its areas of
functioning. Identifying family strengths that appear to increase positive

functioning may be the key to supporting and building family coping resources (Rivara, Jaffe, Polissar, Fay, Liao, & Martin (1996). All the above factors, moreover, rarely occur together, and successful adjustment may take place without all of them.

INTERVENTIONS

Emerging from many of the issues discussed in this chapter is the demand for appropriate interventions by health professionals and parents. Cohen (1999) also suggests that interventions with disabled children should activate family resources if resilience among family members is to be promoted. Specific strategies such as putting the illness in its place, and "seeing the whole child in the whole picture" (p. 158) may encourage managing the illness in the context of total family life. Weihs, Fisher, and Baird (2002) report that the most common type of family-focused intervention for the management of chronic disease in children and adolescents is psychoeducational. But it is important that family interventions also be directed toward increases in self-care in accordance with the young person's development. In earlier research with family members affected by traumatic brain injury, Pieper (1991) and Pieper and Singer (1991) identified many effective interventions and categorized them into the following areas:

Communication

Communication between parents and professionals, for example, should be characterized by honest and concrete explanations emphasizing descriptions, not interpretations. When talking with siblings, their developmental level must be considered. Words have different meanings for children at different ages. A child may perceive a sense of time differently. For example, "soon" many mean tomorrow to the child, but "not this week" to the adult. Further, communication should be encouraged between the parents of the young person's friends as well as peers regarding the symptoms of the disability or chronic illness (Miller, 1995).

Expression of Feelings

Children of all ages must be given the opportunity to express their feelings. Siblings, as well as the young person with a disability, are grieving in their own way over perceived losses. To handle anger and frustration, older and even younger children might be encouraged to release their feelings about what is happening in their lives in constructive ways, such as with drawings or a journal. Younger children might be encouraged to tell a story about a friend in order to express some of their ideas or feelings.

Support:

While parents are indispensable for the life development of their offspring, other adults and significant others can also be important resources for their children. These adults may also become friends who can share in the emotional support and growth of children. Support also includes available counseling, a descriptive and directive type of intervention which focuses on what is happening here and now and how it can be managed. Groups may be more cost-effective and have a greater impact when they provide information and shared care-giving experiences. However, as with individual counseling, group interventions should be approached cautiously by carefully exploring the skills of the group leader and the guidelines for confidentiality. Sibling support groups can also be quite helpful since they offer young people an opportunity to express concerns and frustrations and get feedback from others.

Each of these three interventions suggests ways for families to balance their needs, interests, and time. They also can result in a balance between medical management, quality of life, and developmental demands of the child and adolescent (Miller, 1995). Adjusting to an illness or disability is a complex challenge for a family, requiring the qualities of flexibility, openness, generosity, and the ability to listen to family members. Communication skills and the willingness to allow family members to appropriately express their feelings and take advantage of available support systems are all possible approaches to assist the family in readjusting on a daily basis to the demands of living with an illness or disability.

CONCLUSION

For family members, educators, and health professionals, it is important to address psychosocial adjustment issues early in the recovery process of children and adolescents with disabilities. Solving the continued difficulties that impact on the family requires an understanding of the complex needs of the young person with a disability and the many ways in which the disability can be managed. However, an important theme in this chapter is the emphasis on adaptive outcomes. These are goals that result from both the strengths of families and the awareness by parents and health professionals that families can survive and even have enriching lives while coping with illness, loss, disability, and change.

The following personal statement by Celia captures the unique journey of a child and her family from the perspective of her mother, who also shares how she copes.

CELIA: A PARENT'S BURDEN AND OPPORTUNITY

My daughter was 11 years old when she was suddenly hit by a car while riding her bicycle on a street near our home. It was a hit-and-run accident. The car sideswiped Celia, knocked her off the bicycle, and then sped away. That was almost 3 years ago, and since then the lives of the family have been changed.

Celia was unconscious for about two hours and had several facial lacerations and broken ribs. The face and ribs have healed, leaving few scars, but it is her brain injury that has caused us the most suffering. Unfortunately, Celia was not wearing her helmet; she had dashed off the porch where she'd been sitting when a friend waved to her to ride with her. When she woke up in the hospital, the doctor stated that he thought it was just a concussion and that she would be fine in a couple of months. But that is not what happened.

When our daughter came home after three days in the hospital, we noticed slight behavioral changes which became more noticeable over time. Normally a very focused, determined child, Celia became easily distracted, quick to lose her temper, and frequently agitated during the day. The accident happened during the summer while Celia was involved in a reading program at the local library. Before the accident, she would love to tell us the stories she had read; afterwards she couldn't remember any of the stories immediately after reading them. Finally, we took her to our family physician, who referred us to a pediatric neurologist. He diagnosed a closed head injury and recommended different treatments focusing on behavioral and cognitive goals.

Much to Celia's anger and disappointment, we decided to keep her out of school for a year after my husband and I realized that the school was not equipped to deal with the combination of behavioral and mind problems. So we went the home-study route, with different therapists helping us with the many problems that kept coming our way.

Has the injury made a difference in our family life? It sure has. Both my husband and I, married now for 19 years, are from Ireland. We met here while I was working as a nanny for a wealthy family and Michael was going to school to become a chemist. Now he has a very good job with the federal government, and when our second child was born, I left my job in the embroidery factory and decided to be a full-time homemaker. Celia is the youngest of our four children and the only girl. Our oldest just graduated from high school, and the other two boys are in a public high school. Unfortu-

nately, my husband is developing a drinking problem, claiming that he is so
terribly upset at what has happened to his only daughter and what kind of
a future she will have. Celia is now back in regular school in the sixth grade,
but has a learning disability and struggles with all of her school subjects.
Before the accident she was the brightest person in the class. It is now a
disappointment, a cloud that we have to live with every day.

Celia's injury has caused problems, but it has also been a learning experience. Her brothers assume many more responsibilities, like making sure her
home and social environment are safe. They have become more vigilant
about the welfare of someone else. Perhaps they are closer to each other, if
adolescent brothers are able to be close with one another. My husband, as
I have mentioned, has not been dealing with all of this very well. I have urged
him to get help with his drinking, but he says he is not ready and he is mad
at God for allowing this to happen to us. Fortunately, he is not abusive to
me or the children. I guess you would call him a "silent drinker," preferring
to carry his sorrow in private and wall himself off from all of us. He now
doesn't do much with the boys, and that is very painful for me.

I think I am managing pretty well. Celia gets frustrated very easily over
her schoolwork, has trouble continuing a conversation, and when there is
loud noise in the house, she becomes very upset, shouting and yelling at us.
A previously quiet girl has become a screamer. But each morning I write
down three goals I wish to accomplish for that day, and this provides a
structure for my daily life. I am very specific about these goals, and part of
this exercise is to identify those stressors in my life. I don't like my friends
to tell me what the stressors are. I should know what is bothering me. Also,
I meet twice a month with a group of parents who have children who are
brain-injured. What a help these people have been. It took awhile to accept
the need for this group. I wasn't ready until I realized that I just didn't know
what to do about behavior and school problems. The group gives me ideas
about how to manage Celia's temper and outbursts and how to deal with my
boys, who at times, I know, feel resentful about so much attention that Celia
receives from us. These people have also become my friends, and without
them the days would be longer and the future might seem really hopeless.

I pray that Celia will learn to manage her difficulties. Prayer, support, and
competent professional intervention are what we have. But there is something
else that I have learned and it is an important part of my dealing with this.
I have become an advocate for my daughter, pleading her cause to her
teachers and health professionals. I am, by nature, a quiet person, but being
shy and unassertive as a parent of a child with a head injury will get me
nowhere. First of all, I don't understand much of the information the doctors
are communicating to me, and I must speak out if I wish to understand what
is going on. The school situation is something else. My daughter needs some
classroom accommodations, and if I am lucky, someone may suggest these
to me. Otherwise, I have to learn what is needed and then go after it. Then
there is the whole issue of discipline. The group I attend has given me some
good ideas, but I have to search for people who are experts in behavioral
management. I am not a leader—just a person who stands up for the rights

of my family and who wishes the best quality of life for our children. And with my advocacy I try to be good to myself. Taking care of yourself is very important. I am not a selfish person, but I look for new activities in which all the family can participate. These new activities bring variety to all of us and give us all some satisfaction. It makes thinking about the unknown future more bearable.

DISCUSSION QUESTIONS

1. Why is a "hit and run" more complicated for a family to deal with?
2. Was the doctor's statement that "she would be fine" helpful or not?
3. Was the family adequately prepared for the changes, manifested by Celia, when she returned home? If not what could have been done to facilitate the transition?
4. Do you think it was better to keep Celia at home rather than have her attend school? What were some other options?
5. Discuss the issues and implications of a child's gender as related to a family's reaction to a brain injury.
6. How should a family member be approached when substance abuse has become a means of coping with a brain injury and a roadblock to adjustment?
7. Do you think that the adjustment to the brain injury of an "average" child is different from that of a brain injury to a "gifted" child?
8. How are religious beliefs manifested in this personal statement?
9. Do you think that the mother is coping well? Are there areas that should be considered and attended to? In the present? The future?
10. Are there any risks to being an advocate?
11. Discuss how roles in the family have changed as a result of Celia's brain injury.

SET 2: WHO SHOULD PAY?

PERSPECTIVE

In addition to the emotional and physical complexity surrounding childhood illness and disability, families must also deal with complex financial realities. If insurance is limited or nonexistent or if large settlements are not viable, families are often forced to turn to other sources of support, which may be limited in scope and impact. At this point, families are forced to reevaluate the situation, and they are often faced with very difficult choices. Often the choices are not who *should* pay, but who *can* pay, who *wants* to pay, and who *is willing* to help.

Exploration

1. If you were in need of significant financial assistance from your family, would they respond? Why or why not?
2. Would you be available on a long-term basis to provide maximum financial assistance for a member of your family who had a brain injury, spinal cord injury, AIDS, or Alzheimer's disease?

REFERENCES

Breakey, J. W. (1997). Body image: The inner mirror. *Journal of Prosthetics and Orthotics, 9*(3), 107–112.

Clarke, E. (1996). Children and adolescents with traumatic brain injury: Reintegration challenges in educational settings. *Journal of Learning Disabilities, 29* (5), 549–551.

Cloutier, P. F., Manion, I. G., Walker, J. G., & Johnson, S. M. (2002). Emotionally focused interventions for couples with chronically ill children: A 2-year follow-up. *Journal of Marital and Family Therapy, 28* (4), 391–398.

Cohen, M. S. (1999). Families coping with childhood chronic illness: A research review. *FamilySystems and Health, 17* (2), 149–163.

Coppa, C., Hepburn, J., Strauss, D., & Yody, B. (1999). Return to home after acquired brain injury: Is the family ready? *Brain Injury Source, 3*, 18–21.

Dahlquist, L. M., Czyzewski, D. I., & Jones, C. L. (1995). Parents of children with cancer: A longitudinal study of emotional distress, coping style, and marital adjustment two and twenty months after diagnosis. *Journal of Pediatric Psychology, 21*, 541–554.

Gaither, R., Bingen, K., & Hopkins, J. (2000). When the bough breaks: The relationship between chronic illness in children and couple functioning. In K. B. Schmaling & T. Goldman Sher (Eds.), *The psychology of couples and illness: Theory, research, and practice*. Washington, DC: American Psychological Association.

Harry, B. (2002). Trends and issues in serving culturally diverse families of children with disabilities. *The Journal of Special Education, 36* (3), 131–138.

Johnson, L. S. (1997). Developmental strategies for counseling the child whose parent or sibling has cancer. *Journal of Counseling and Development, 75*, 417–427.

Lustig, D. C. (2002). Family coping in families with a child with a disability. *Education and Training in Mental Retardation and Developmental Disabilities, 37* (1), 14–22.

Miller, B. (1995). Promoting healthy function and development in chronically ill children: A primary care approach. *Family Systems and Medicine, 13*, 187–200.

Nixon, C. L., & Cummings, E. (1999). Sibling disability and children's reactivity to conflicts involving family members. *Journal of Family Psychology, 13* (2), 274–285.

Patrick, P. D., & Hostler, S. L. (1998). Neurobehavioral outcomes after acquired brain injury in childhood. *Brain Injury Source*, 2, 26–31.

Patterson, J. M. (1988). Chronic illness in children and the impact on families. In C. S. Chilman, E. W. Nunnally, & F. M. Cox (Eds.), *Chronic illness and disability*. Newbury Park, CA: Sage Publications.

Patterson, J. M., Garwick, A. W., Bennett, F. C., & Blum, R. W. (1997). Social support in families of children with chronic conditions: Supportive and nonsupportive behaviors. *Journal of Developmental and Behavioral Pediatrics, 18* (6), 383–392.

Patterson, J. M., & Garwick, A. (1998). Coping with chronic illness: A family systems perspective on living with diabetes. In G. Werther & J. Court (Eds.), *Diabetes and the adolescent.*Melbourne, Australia: Miranova Publishing.

Pieper, B. (1991). *In home family supports: What families of youngsters with traumatic brain injury really need*. Albany, NY: New York State Head Injury Association.

Pieper, B., & Singer, G. (1991). *Model family partnerships for interventions in children with traumatic brain injury*. Albany, NY: New York State Head Injury Association.

Rivara, J. M., Jaffe, K. M., Polissar, N. L., Fay, G. S., Liao, S., & Martin, K. M. (1996). Predictors of family functioning and change 3 years after traumatic brain injury in children, *Archives of Physical Medicine and & Rehabilitation*, 79, 90–103.

Smart, J. (2001). Disability, society, and the individual. Gaithersburg, MD: Aspen Publishers, Inc.Varni, J. W., Rapoff, M. A., Waldron, S. A., Gragg, R. A., Bernstein, B. H., & Lindsley, C. B. (1996). Effects of perceived stress on pediatric chronic pain. *Journal of Behavioral Medicine, 19*, 515–528.

Weihs, K., Fisher, L., & Baird, M. (2002). Families, health, and behavior. *Family Systems and health, 20* (1), 7–46.

3

Impact of Illness and Disability on Adults

With advances in medical and assistive technology and improvements in pharmacological interventions, more people are physically surviving severe disabilities and chronic illness. But the emotional and behavioral responses emerging from these experiences are ever-present and continuing realities. These reactions can influence how the individual will adapt, and also can affect the family's process and outcome of adjustment. Intense and problematic emotions from a family member who is severely disabled or chronically ill may prevent the family from extending help that could be directed to meeting rehabilitation goals. If a person is continually angry about his or her limitations consequent to a severe disability or illness, then this emotion will frequently be projected onto others, creating an atmosphere of tension and anxiety. A family member who refuses to participate in prescribed therapies claiming, "I don't have a problem with that," or "The problems are just too overwhelming," will cause frustration and disappointment within the family system. It is important to note, however, that intense emotions are often very appropriate given the intensity of the loss.

The increased survival rate among those who have been severely injured or diagnosed with a severe illness has facilitated the emergence of new treatment approaches, many of which emphasize the productive functioning of the total person after the injury (Marinelli & Dell Orto, 1999). Although adult survivors have unique problems and vary in their emotional and behavioral responses, an understanding of these reactions can play a key role in their functioning. If optimum treatment and rehabilitation are to be achieved, an awareness of both the individual effects of illness and disability and of the determining factors in the person's response is necessary. Determinants are guideposts for understanding individual reactions. This chapter will describe such determinants, as well as the distinctive needs caused by the different reactions and the adaptive tasks associated with the family members' attempts to adjust to the severe disability or chronic illness.

To be noted is that individual and family emotional reactions to major life losses and changes, e.g., illness and disability, are not static, but more developmental. In other words, an individual with a disability or chronic illness may show specific responses because of certain stages in the recovery and rehabilitation process. After discharge from in-hospital rehabilitation care, for example, a person may display enthusiastic hope for complete recovery and denial of any long-term limitations or further decline. As the expectation of full recovery by a person with severe impairment becomes less and less realistic over time, a specific emotion or combination of emotions may dominate this individual's behavior, such as performance anxiety, defensiveness, and/or confusion. A lingering hope may later give way to quiet desperation and angry outbursts with the gradual acknowledgement that certain effects will probably be permanent (e.g., limitations from stroke and spinal cord injury) or get worse (e.g., multiple sclerosis and Alzheimer's disease), and new adjustments and adaptations are required.

Besides specific recovery stages, however, there are other determinants to a person's reaction to a disability or chronic illness, many of which are:

1. *Triggering events.* There is usually a difference in how one reacts to a disability if the onset was sudden or was the result, for example, of the aging process. An accident or an act of violence resulting in a severe injury may cause shock, confusion, anger, and guilt. The aging process does not necessarily convey the expectation that a severe physical or mental limitation is expected, but the element of surprise and shock may not be as intense as from an unexpected disruption in daily functioning. Responses, though, are very individual and often depend on a person's frame of reference regarding life and living. Issues of blame, moreover, often are associated with triggering event. Blame then produces unique expression of anger and resentment. A severe disability caused by a hit and run or an uninsured driver can generate continued blame and intense anger.

2. *Severity and type of illness or disability.* Whether the severe disability is visible or not, what body parts are affected, and how seriously the disability or illness affects such functions as mobility, seeing, hearing, communication, and sexuality will all influence the response of an individual and his or her family (Rolland, 1994). Disfigurement may cause isolation and withdrawing behavior. The

loss of certain abilities to perform many expected functions may prompt reactions of anger and anxiety. Emotional withdrawal from family and friends and affective disturbances such as radical mood swings and depression can be caused by the severity of the injury. At this time the power and impact of positive role models become a vital force in treatment and rehabilitation.

3.   *Personal influences.* There are several determinants that emerge primarily from the individual who is experiencing the chronic illness or disability:

   A.   *Perceived threats.* Being chronically ill or severely disabled involves threats to an individual's self-concept, values, belief systems, and commitments to family, work, and social roles. The intensity and kind of threats depends on the person's perceptions and perhaps the risks involved during treatment and initial adjustment phases. If a family member perceives, for example, that his/her severe illness or disability will disrupt or terminate customary social roles and activities, then this individual may feel angry, isolated, and alienated, and may become withdrawn or motivated to change their family role within the context of this new situation.

   B.   *Personality resources/style.* If someone is accustomed to being dependent on others for most daily needs and has always been reluctant to show initiative or independent behavior, that person may react to an illness or disability by becoming even more dependent than before the injury onset. If individuals view themselves as mentally alert, vigorous, sexually active, independent, and physically strong, then a disability may cause heightened feelings of vulnerability, depression, and hopelessness. Other factors included in personality resources are self-esteem, motivation, confidence in one's strengths, and positive, learned behavior from past experiences. Previous life experiences may have assisted the person to learn more adaptable ways to adjust to a new loss or access new opportunities (Weihs, Fisher, & Baird, 2002). Also, if an individual had the continued satisfaction of competence in handling many life tasks, and emotional needs have been achieved, feelings of adequacy and empowerment may gradually return post-trauma. However, due to a perceived or real depletion of personality resources, dealing with a prior crisis does not mean that the person can cope with a new and unique experience that may have dramatically changed his or her world and the ability to enjoy life as it is newly emerging.

Personality style, in the context of loss, illness, and disability refers more to attitudes of optimism and pessimism and beliefs and values about how one controls the events emerging from a medical trauma than specific behaviors used to manage its personal and social effects. If someone has the conviction, for example, that he/she can somehow "master" the situation and not rely solely on external influences, then this belief may generate feelings of competence. An optimistic attitude, moreover, may stimulate feelings of hope that enable a family member to negotiate appropriately an indefinite post-trauma period that may be demanding and quite overwhelming (Bader & Robbins, 2001). It may be a long time before symptom stability is achieved, and for individuals who are accustomed to having a measure of control over such life events as health, career, and family life, living with the unknown and episodic occurrences of symptoms may bring continued anxiety, distress, irritability, and impatience. These feelings may be ameliorated or contained by hope and optimism.

C.   *Body image.* The body and the mind reflect who we are, were, or want to be. Under the best of circumstances, most people are engaged in a constant struggle trying to improve their body, its function, or its appearance (Breakey, 1997). Following a trauma the body and the mind may be changed in a way that is not acceptable to the person or those who are important to them, e.g., family, spouse, significant others, employers, etc. If someone's identity revolves around specific capabilities of the body, e.g., an athlete, or one's livelihood depends on a certain function, e.g., playing the piano, then loss of the capability or function could be emotionally devastating to the impaired individual. As a person with spinal cord injury stated, however, "There are many things I can still do. I miss what was but I am learning to enjoy what is and what can be."

D.   *Religion/philosophy of life.* Values rooted in religion or a personal philosophy are for many persons guideposts for integrity and purposeful living (Boswell, Knight, Hamer, & McChesney, 2001). For varied reasons a person may feel that the illness or disability is a punishment for past sins or a unique opportunity to practice one's beliefs. Or one may believe that the acceptance of loss often associated with a chronic illness or disability is an opportunity to meet a spiri-

tual challenge. Drawing from spiritual resources may alleviate
feelings of anguish caused by the medical situation and encourage hope. This hope may facilitate a more optimistic
attitude, which identifies the personal gains accruing from
pain and loss (Longo & Peterson, 2002).

E. *The life stage of the person.* People go through many life stages
as they age and develop. The time of onset of illness or
disability in the life cycle is particularly important. Many
disabilities occur in the prime of life, a period when certain
interpersonal and occupational tasks should be accomplished
that will have a direct impact on the person's future and
options. Often someone has just begun a new career. When
the injury occurs at a time when a person has great expectations, the emotional reaction could be more severe. For example, a 21-year-old unmarried man or woman living with his
or her parents may experience a major trauma at a time
when college graduation or a significant job promotion is
approaching. The impairment/disability often results in a
disruption in life plans. This disruption can be more complicated if an adult child becomes disabled, is abandoned by a
spouse, and returns home to live with elderly parents trying
to cope with their own issues related to aging and frail health.

F. *Culture.* A person's culture can make a difference in how he
or she responds to a severe illness or disability (Cohen, 1999).
Decision-making strategies and support resources are often
culturally determined (Harry, 2002). Also, different ethnic
groups have distinctive health-belief models, and their relationships to health professionals are influenced by these beliefs (Santana & Santana, 2001; Stanhope, 2002). In turn,
the manner of decision making for varied problems arising
during treatment and rehabilitation may alleviate anxiety;
available and supportive extended family members may provide needed comfort during the difficult times of treatment
and adjustment to disability-related limitations.

G. *Role changes.* Each family member usually has designated roles
within family life. But when a disability or chronic illness
causes role ambiguity, conflict, or strain, then feelings of
frustrations, anxiety, and disappointment may result. If the
primary wage earner within the family suddenly becomes
unemployed, then stress is created among family members.
The feelings of frustration, vulnerability, and disappointment
can overwhelm this family member who must adjust to a new

family role. If a wife and mother has to undergo regular medical treatments because of chronic illness, then this constant involvement may cause persistent conflict when attempting to perform her home responsibilities. Conflict stimulates stress and induces anxiety and frustration, as well as creating opportunities for new beginnings.

4.   *Contextual influences.* There are several determinants emerging from the individual's living and working environment that may cause a positive or negative response to the loss and illness/disability experience.

    A.   *Family reactions.* Family members can have a profound influence on how individuals will react to their chronic illness or disability (Cohen, 1999; Weihs, Fisher, & Baird, 2002). Economic and relationship changes within the family result from dealing with a future that may be perceived as threatening. Issues of blame and resentment often surface in the family system. If the disability was caused by carelessness or neglect, family members may harbor continued feelings of blame toward the person with the disability or the person responsible, especially if the family's future plans are seriously disrupted or financial losses are severe. When the person with a disability recognizes these attitudes, guilt feelings accompanied by frustration and depression often emerge. Also, unrealistic expectations concerning responses to adaptive or treatment demands may foster feelings of inadequacy, uncertainty, and desperation. Moreover, unfinished business around issues of unresolved anger may create a family atmosphere of tension (Lane, 1995). The stress accompanying this tension may be another factor that the person with an illness or disability has to deal with in his or her adjustment efforts. As a wife said to her husband, "You must get better. I am too young to be married to an invalid."

    After the initial shock caused by the trauma subsides, families may begin to experience or develop a positive reaction to the severe illness or disability. Communication patterns among family members may improve, and family roles become clearer as well as more realistic expectations emerge. These family dynamics create an environment where accommodations to treatment and rehabilitation demands are made with accepting attitudes. In turn, the family member who has a severe disability/illness finds an atmosphere characterized more by support and understanding than isolation and rejection. This support facilitates the difficult journey of the person and family to a more successful treatment and adjustment (Weihs, Fisher, & Baird, 2002).

B.   *Timing and type of therapeutic intervention.* Appropriate early intervention "sets the stage" for someone to focus more on the residual assets than the limitations of an illness or disability. Such attention can be most challenging during times of intense adjustment that may require moving beyond what was toward what can be. Medical care is necessarily directed to treating the problems, and those strengths and remaining capacities may be lost in the perception of what has happened and what has been lost or changed. But an emerging perspective on the positive potential could help to minimize a lingering depression, encourage a process of coping, and stimulate one's motivation to resume, as much as possible, former life activities. It is not only early intervention, however, which can make a difference in a person's emotional reaction. The attitudes of health professionals and how they communicate information about illness and disability when providing treatment and rehabilitation can have a decided impact on an individual. A physician or nurse who only emphasizes what one cannot do instead of one's residual abilities may be inadvertently undermining that person's hope. As noted earlier, role models can make a difference in the future vision a person has regarding choices to be made.

C.   *Institutional supports.* These supports can include many forms of assistance provided by employment, professional service, and academic arenas. When these resources communicate a positive, realistic attitude to what has happened and to what can be, and provide appropriate support for the family and the member who is chronically ill or severely disabled, then this can make all the difference to the individual who may be struggling to understand and manage what has happened and what will be. A person's hope is stimulated or nurtured by such support. In contrast, an indifferent attitude may only add to the individual's anxiety, depression, aloneness, and feelings of worthlessness. For many persons, identity is based on their professional career and paid employment and when a sudden life change occurs, usually they anticipate support from an area to which they have devoted so much time. When such support exists, it is a contributing factor to eventual disability or illness adjustment; when the support is absent, it can be devastating and often undermines any enthusiasm for adaptation (Martz, 2002).

5. *Stigma and societal reactions.* Certain mental and physical illnesses cause discriminating response reactions formed around stereotypes and misinformation. If someone with a severe illness or disability is aware of such negative attitudes, then this person may feel alienated or marginalized or devalued. Also, the visibility of certain disabilities and their accompanying unique behaviors may arouse fear or anxiety in others. In turn, the person with the disability may feel awkward and also anxious in social relationships. An individual's perception of being negatively viewed or devalued only aggravates a lingering depression. Anger may also result from this perception. Both of these emotions can be obstacles along the path to adjustment (Lane, 1995) But a focus on self-determination can become a counterbalance to negative influences outside the person and the family.

Illness and disability do not occur in a vacuum. Personal and contextual influences have a significant impact on how one is going to react to the changes and losses accompanying and consequent to illness or disability. Adaptation to an individual's new limitations and newly discovered assets may necessitate learning new skills and exploring new opportunities. But when a person is aware of what is causing a specific emotional response or behavior, then the beginning step can be taken in this learning and adaptation process. Another step in this process is an understanding of how one is responding to a chronic illness or severe disability. Such knowledge provides a guideline to what can be done to assist in the individual's adjustment. The following section identifies these reactions.

PSYCHOSOCIAL REACTION TO ILLNESS AND DISABILITY

The issues related to an individual's emotional response and eventual adjustment to a severe illness or disability have been a focus of the clinical and research literature and subject to conceptual disagreements and clinically opposed views (Livneh, 2001; Shontz, 1978). One area of discussion has been the progression of phases leading to adaptation. The majority of models acknowledge the existence of a series, stages, or progression of reactions individually experienced that may be short or longterm (Kendall & Buys, 1998; Kübler-Ross, 1969; Pearson, 1973; Power & Dell Orto, 1980; Weisman, 1972). These responses can occur immediately following the onset of a disability (denial and shock), at an intermediate stage (grief, depression, anger), and late or longerterm (many of which involve acceptance, accommodation, and adaptation to the reactions of continued dependency and feelings of helplessness and hopelessness) (Livneh, 2001). Though there is disagreement about the total number of stages in the adjustment process to illness or disability, most response models describe an initial period of shock and/or denial, which is followed by significant distress, and usually concludes with acceptance of one's situation (Kendall & Buys, 1998; Power, Dell Orto, & Gibbons, 1988; Weisman, 1972).

While most individuals show a general trend towards a positive adjustment to a severe disability over an indefinite period of time, Kendall and Buys (1998) believe that stage models have a number of negative implications for the rehabilitation process. These models of adjustment tend to normalize responses such as denial and distress following acquired disability, or are purely descriptive and provide little information about what contributes to individual differences in the adjustment process, or finally, do not adequately match the subjective experience of people with acquired disability (Yoshida, 1993). Individuals may also vary in how they move through the adjustment process. There is the tendency, moreover, to view reactive stage models as a process of socialization into the "role" of a person with a disability (Kendall & Buys, 1998).

While there are limitations to the stage models, they do provide suggested guidelines to what an individual may be emotionally experiencing when responding to a severe, medical condition. Importantly, the process of psychosocial adjustment following acquired disability can be a continuous life transition rather than a time-limited one. A person may constantly struggle with chronic sorrow, anger, and anxiety over perceived losses. Consequently, adaptation may be recurrent (Kendall & Buys, 1998), and specific emotions are likely to re-emerge at regular intervals. This is especially so with medical conditions which involve remission and exacerbation, such as multiple sclerosis and cancer (Coyle & Halper, 2001).

What may influence the recurrent nature of psychosocial adjustment is the person's periodic awareness of personal resources to deal with events associated with the demands of treatment, rehabilitation and other daily responsibilities. Or an individual may be searching for a meaning to what has happened to them personally as a result of the disability/illness, and may be seeking ways to have some control over an certain or uncertain future, e.g., conditions that improve, deteriorate, or are terminal. Such seeking and searching may be stressful, is often confusing, and a person may emotionally shift from feelings of self-acceptance to self-rejection (Barnard, 1990). This shift will also trigger different reactive emotions that may have occurred earlier in the reactive process.

Putting aside the debate over the validity of adjustment models to severe illness/disability, there are certain themes that are evident across the lives of individuals living with and recovering from the experience. These themes are:

1. *Denial of the implications of the trauma.* Denial may include minimization of any personal threat, existence of negative emotion, loss of cognitive and/or physical abilities, or the possibility that one will not completely recover. For example, denial in the person experiencing the effects of brain injury may take the form of denying past abilities or current limitations, pushing oneself too hard, and an unwillingness to give up control, identity, and value in the eyes of self and others (Armstrong, 1991). Deaton (1986) reports that denying past abilities may result in avoidance of grief, failure to participate in rehabilitation, and lack of motivation. Acting as though present status is identical to pre-injury status may also result in a failure to remediate deficits and alienation of family and friends. Deaton further explains that pushing oneself too hard can cause physical injuries and depression.

Denial can also serve an adaptive purpose for it can allow the individual to maintain a sense of self-esteem, reduce stress, and possibly generate encouragement and hope (Livneh, Martz, & Wilson, 2001). Because of denial, the person with a disability can control, insofar as the individual as the capacity to do so, his or her perception of the trauma and emotional reaction to it (Matt, Sementilli, & Burish, 1988). All in all, however, although denial may reduce immediate distress, it frequently has a detrimental long-term effect (Watson, Green, Blake, & Schrapnell, 1984). If a person does not finally acknowledge the limitations caused by the illness or disability, then the recovery process may be slowed considerably, and little remediation of living deficits can occur. This is especially true if standard methods of treatment are ignored. The person may increase the risk for further limitations, e.g., refusing to accept that hypertension exists or believes that the lump will go away.

2. *Grieving over perceived losses.* For some persons living with a demanding illness or disability, grief is a profound sadness or sorrow due to the significant changes or reduction in such areas as health, independence, sense of control over life, established roles inside the home, sexuality, familiar daily routine, and means of productivity. Family members mourn the person who was there before the trauma. Importantly, grief is so many little deaths along the way of recovery and/

or possible adjustment. These deaths continue to occur as the individual realizes that selected life functions may not be restored, and one has to come to terms with the eventual possibility of little or no return to pre-injury capacities (Lewis, 1983). The grieving may be further characterized by the persistent desire for recovery of lost abilities, or the need to express negative feelings because of many losses and the inability to do so (Brown, 1990). The grief is often accompanied by feelings of anger and helplessness, and anger is often directed toward others (Lane, 1995). While it is appropriate to grieve it is important to create a process that facilitates grief resolution so that new beginnings can be made.

3.   *Guilt.* Guilt is better understood in the context of interpersonal relationships. For example, family members may often express to the person with a disability their beliefs about why the trauma occurred, such as not wearing a seatbelt or a motorcycle helmet. This blaming type of communication often results in feelings of guilt that include inadequacy, shame, sadness, agitation, self-condemnation, and anger. It may be extremely difficult for the family and significant others to accept the reality of what has happened, and consequently they deal with their feelings by blaming the injured or ill person for all the changes. This may result in thwarting the grief process and not moving on.

4.   *Social isolation.* Though identified as a significant behavior that accompanies depression, decreased social contact and the disruption of friendships post-trauma may facilitate a period of social isolation. The isolation can also represent a recovery period for individuals who need time to marshal their resources and deal with adjustment issues. Many persons further believe that they have lost their primary identity as an individual, whether it is as a parent, wage earner, lover, or athlete. Separating oneself temporarily from accustomed friends may provide an opportunity to reflect on what steps are needed to recapture a semblance of that former identity. This period of re-evaluation also includes the identification of personal resources that can be utilized in restarting one's life.

The issues of preserving or rebuilding social relationships were addressed earlier in research by Betty Cogswell (1968). Though she has written primarily about the resocialization process with persons who have a spinal cord injury, often a similar re-socialization may occur with persons who have other severe illnesses or disabilities, especially if the disability or illness is stigmatized or evokes a particular stereotypical response about residual capabilities. In particular, during outpatient treatment, the individual may be cautious in the selection of social opportunities, and when possible, he or she will carefully choose settings that have frequently been used, and may only associate with long-time friends. Because he or she eventually realizes the extent of physical, cognitive, and emotional limitations, and goes through a period of readjustment in perception of self-confidence, remaining abilities, and realistic opportunities, the person with an illness or disability may be hesitant about involvement in any new life plans, associations, or even career opportunities. Such cautiousness is a reflection of feelings of vulnerability and "being different". On the other hand, a consequence of the medical condition could be a very different reaction and the person could replace caution with impulsiveness, and engage in decision making that is more problematic than helpful.

5. *Anger.* Though identified earlier as a component of other emotional responses to a severe illness and disability, anger is often a dominant response to a medical trauma, especially when the event or diagnosis is unexpected. Combined with the actual limitations caused by the severe disability/chronic illness, society imposes additional limitations through the lack of equal access to such resources as financial, employment, education, recreation, and social opportunities. Individuals may believe they lack the ability to utilize fully these resources, and consequently may substitute anger for feelings of weakness (Lane, 1995). A family member becomes frustrated over perceived limitations and the restrictions they may impose, and the emotional response to frustration is anger. As an emotion it can be expressed by silence, moodiness, withdrawal, and guilt. Anger can also be projected onto other family members and friends by unnecessary arguing, continued sarcasm, and constant criticism.

Anger is also caused by the person's awareness of the pain and vulnerability usually associated with loss. The loss of dreams and expectations, promising opportunities, and looking towards an uncertain future may stimulate feelings of inadequacy and powerlessness which generate and feed the emotion of anger. As one's choices become more limited, an individual becomes frustrated as benefits that others take for granted become elusive. Anger may be an attempt to regain some choices, freedom, and autonomy (Lane, 1995).

Yet, many persons who are experiencing a serious medical condition may, after a period of personal adjustment, use anger for creative purposes. It can become a constructive tool for communicating clearly and honestly what one needs. Anger may motivate one's resolve to achieve treatment and rehabilitation goals expeditiously.

6. *Depression.* Though Freud saw depression as anger turned inward (Campbell, 1986), with the many losses associated with severe disability

and illness, depression is not simply "anger turned inward" (Martin, 1986). While closely connected and at times feeding on one another, anger and depression may be learned coping strategies used to defend one against many anxieties and fears emerging from the disability experience (Glazer, Emery, Frid, & Banyasz, 2002; Lane, 1995). A persistent sad or empty mood and withdrawing from many customary activities may be a way to buffer oneself against the feelings of vulnerability and bitterness arising from perceived frustrations and losses (Miller, 2002). But people who are truly depressed can rarely achieve acceptance of a loss (O'Connor, 1997). In depression, moreover, there is a gradual numbing of feelings and often a suppression of impulses or unwanted emotions. Such feelings of loneliness and disappointment are silently experienced as the varied losses affect a person's life.

Most people, when becoming aware of their responses to their disability or illness, do not actually experience what is called a "clinical depression". Of course some do, but a family member coming to grips with the many disability or illness-induced changes usually harbors intense feelings of sadness and helplessness. Yet the necessary activities of daily life are still being pursued while the individual adjusts to new limitations and changed expectations. At times it is a fine line between a significant depression and periodic sadness and anxiety with someone who may have eating and sleep disturbances, feelings of pessimism and worthlessness, and diminished ability to make decisions, but who at the same time is appropriately responding to treatment and rehabilitation demands, is motivated to adapt to the medical condition, and attempts to maintain an energy level to meet, as much as possible, family responsibilities. People who are experiencing a depression resulting from severe illness or disability induced losses may go through the motions of eating, sex, work, or play, but the activities seem hollow. Those with more severe depressions withdraw from these activities, feeling too tired or tense to participate (O'Connor, 1997).

7. *Coping styles.* Individuals with a major illness or disability will adapt selected coping mechanisms that represent styles for dealing with the perceived losses (Bader & Robbins, 2001). They are defense strategies necessary for dealing with the difficult demands associated with a severe medical condition. Coping styles can often be creative and adaptive, or they can be used to distort reality or to drive a wedge between an experience and a feeling. Distortion is a form of denial, and avoiding an expected emotion accompanying the medical condition is a form of isolation. Both denial and isolation can be used for adaptive purposes, as stated earlier in this chapter. They may allow the family member to keep a more accurate perspective on what is happening, and allow this individual to maintain self-esteem.

Coping may also include (1) displacement—anger over what one has lost may be displaced among relatives, friends, or others; (2) regression—reverting to past methods of gaining gratification, as when one formerly self-reliant person becomes extremely dependent; and (3) intellectualization—belief, especially if one is older, that "I have lived a full life . . . it could have been much worse . . . perhaps I now will become a better person" (Brown, 1990).

Coping styles include the varied modes of dealing with the challenges ranging from pain, perceived losses, an uncertain future, redirection of goals, and relationship changes. Coping styles can be more problem-focused, such as seeking information and support, or emotion-focused, such as releasing anger or accepting the situation with resignation. These coping styles are constantly changing cognitive and behavioral efforts to manage specific external and internal demands which are viewed as taxing the resource of the person with an illness or disability (Matt, Sementilli, & Burish, 1988).

8. *Acceptance.* Acceptance is more of an active "state," a process characterized by continual mental decisions to live with the realities of the losses associated with severe illness or disability but still harboring ambivalent feelings about one's personal future. The response is not necessarily a resignation to all that has happened, yet a time when an individual has adapted to a new mode of living and is still struggling with recurrent feelings of anger, blame, denial, and helplessness. However, these feelings are generally managed as the family member attempts to regain some measure of self-esteem and personal efficacy. With acceptance there is a recognition of limitations that gradually facilitates an appropriate life adjustment that includes gaining a new perspective on living. An individual with a severe illness or disability begins to see that quality of life does not depend totally on what has been lost and even a greatly altered life may be positively handled. New satisfactions or capacities replace, when possible, those that have been lost, and old relationships are renegotiated based on new realities; some will be given up and new ones will be formed. The "state" of acceptance includes the gradual process of redefining the self through new interactions.

NEEDS AND TASKS

Each of the emotional responses of a person and family to loss, change, illness, and disability stimulates specific needs for that individual. Each need becomes another guidepost for ongoing intervention, and if the needs are ignored, then an appropriate adjustment may be delayed or lost entirely. Also, a person's reaction may be shaped by certain tasks that emerge as one goes through the reactive process. These needs and tasks are briefly identified below:

NEEDS

- To search for meaning in the experienced losses
- To seek support, including a "listening ear"
- For validation and respect that "I am still a worthwhile human being"
- For information that may help to manage or reduce uncertainties, meet treatment responsibilities, and minimize the impact of the loss
- To balance treatment or rehabilitation responsibilities with the demands of life roles

TASKS

- To achieve some adjustment to negative events and realities that result from the medical condition
- To maintain a self-image in spite of the assaults on personal, post illness/disability identity (Kendall & Buys, 1998)
- To maintain an emotional equilibrium by avoiding being overcome by periodic, emotional states
- To maintain satisfying social relationships

CULTURAL CONSIDERATIONS

When attempting to understand a person's emotional response to a severe illness or disability, the context in which these reactions occur must be recognized (Harry, 2002). A person's culture, with its norms, values, and expectations, shape one's response to what has occurred, and even mediates an understanding of any problems emerging from the individual's reaction. An identification of the person's culture is particularly important when identifying determinants to a particular response (Stanhope, 2002). Many ethnic groups, for example, follow culturally prescribed standards of achievement in family and occupational spheres (Kim-Rupaow, 2001). When a severe disability or illness is diagnosed, intense anxiety may result in the individual because of the perceived failure to meet these standards. These anxieties may complicate a person's adjustment to the disability/illness induced losses.

Kinship patterns and culturally based rituals, however, may diminish the intensity of a person's response to a sudden loss or life-threatening diagnosis. Family rules for decision making that are culturally based may nourish feelings of acceptance and self-worth. Post-disability identity development may be encouraged by the support structures expected in certain ethnic groups. On the other hand, culturally prescribed gender roles that are too confining may become stumbling blocks to recapturing self-esteem and feelings of personal value. Culture is a silent determinant to an individual's response to severe, medical conditions, and should always be considered in assessment and intervention approaches.

CONCLUSION

Personality and emotional disruptions have a decided impact on the life adjustment of those with a severe illness or disability. During the reactive process, individuals usually seek or are forced to redefine themselves. But this is a cyclic process, as one confronts new challenges and demands associated with the changing treatment and rehabilitation features of the medical condition. The reactive process is also a unique one for individuals. Some persons will cope more successfully than others. Some will have more available coping resources than others, thus stimulating a more effective adaptation to limitations and other perceived losses.

With an understanding of the complexity of illness and disability, the individual, the family, and the health professional are better able to approach life demands from a perspective based on hope tempered by reality. From this frame of reference, effective interventions can be designed that may help persons and their families live more adaptively with the realities of loss and change and the other challenges and opportunities of life and living.

ALINA: BEYOND MS

The following personal statement poignantly illustrates the reaction of one woman to her disability and chronic illness. It highlights the cyclical nature of how one reacts emotionally to a life-changing diagnosis, and the need for support to cope with what cannot be changed.

I began to experience multiple sclerosis symptoms at the age of 31, after graduating with a master's degree in counseling, and just a few days before starting a new job as a child-adolescent therapist at a mental health clinic. At that time, and after several years of marriage, I was also planning on starting a family of two or three children, but MS appeared in my life like a dark cloud that robs you of your light. I became sick, felt defective, and became deeply distressed by blurred vision and numbness. I was deprived of the power to feel. My palms felt cold, as they had lost their warmth. What is it like to feel sick, to feel defective, to feel numb?

Multiple sclerosis brings anger and fear to the diagnosed person. There is experienced anxiety as the person is never free from the disease. When envisioning the future, there is the anticipation of losses. MS can change habits, rearrange priorities and demand sacrifices. I asked myself "What is it like to live with a chronic illness? What is it like to be forced to change habits and priorities? What is it like to live in a shadow, to feel vulnerable, to be wounded? What is it like to live in uncertainty? What is it like to become sick?" The person with MS struggles and engages in a battle against the intrusion of a demonic or malevolent presence into the body. There is the experience of feeling wounded, vulnerable, and liable to succumb. Living with MS means living in a shadow where I do not let others see my true reflection and thus the reflection of pain and fear becomes invisible.

MS has had a profound impact in my life. It is best to describe the experiences related to living with MS by reflecting and writing about it. As I have lived through multiple flare-ups, I have not only experienced a hardening of the tissue, but also of the heart. Flare-ups fill me with bitterness and despair. As lesions invade my mind, I change, remain, and endure. Living with MS is difficult. It is living on pills to treat the symptoms so that I can look OK and function OK. It is hiding the invisible symptoms so others do not see who you are and what you have. Disclosing the illness is significant. It means getting exposed by removing a cover and the secret is made know to others.

Exposing myself brings anxiety and fear, as I taste the bitterness of having a chronic illness. Would the people who know the "healthy me" feel disappointed if they got to know the other me—the me with MS? What is it like to reveal myself to others? What is it like to reveal vulnerable aspects of the self? Multiple sclerosis and its invisible symptoms such as headaches, vertigo, nausea, blurred vision, physical numbness, neck pain, fatigue, and anxiety impose limitations. These limitations can be alleviated when I rest. But what is it like to have to rest when your mind wants to race?

As I feel angry for my fate, I struggle with my faith. Where is God? I do not ask the "why me?" question because it implies that I may approve of someone else having MS. Instead, I ask, "How is it that people have to suffer? What is it like to have faith in God and feel betrayed by an illness?" I go from feeling sad during relapses to feeling overjoyed during remissions. It is difficult to have a sense of contentment when experiencing physical and emotional discomfort, but then, "Would we know comfort if we did not journey through the experience of suffering and pain?" (Buttorff, 1991, p. 238).

There is an "accumulation of knowledge" through lived experiences (Buttorff, 1991). Could we infer that we accumulate knowledge through pain and suffering? What is it like to accumulate knowledge? I have learned about compassion, pain, priorities, forgiveness, acceptance, and unconditional love. As my body (my vision, brain, and spine) continues to be damaged, I remain strong in my determination of continuing my journey through life. As my health deteriorates, I heal. Does the human body have the capacity for self-repair or could it be God is the healer? After all, God is omnipotent, originator and ruler of the universe, a being of supernatural powers or attributes. For some people faith is the invisible force that helps them feel better. What is it like to have faith? What is it like living in this tension?

Yesterday, someone asked me if I was planning on having another child. This time I did not keep my secret about the reason for choosing not to have another child. Instead I searched for the truth and found something lost that I had concealed. I revealed myself to a stranger. As pregnancy seems to have no impact on the mother with MS, delivery seems to precipitate the progression of the illness.

But having MS means that sooner or later you begin treatment. I started receiving weekly intramuscular injections (Avonex) in 1996. I had been treated with steroids that kept me awake at night and hungry all the time. My weeks do not have seven days because of the side effects of Avonex. I feel sick with flu-like symptoms for a day or two. Symptoms that get me into bed, symptoms that get me to rest. I feel tense—bruises below my shoulder are my weekly tattoos. Yesterday my husband gave me the weekly shot. There was a rush of fear, anxiety, and anger as I anticipate the thick, long needle penetrating my skin. My arms hurt from too many shots—four years behind me and many years to go.

Duval (1984) writes about the psychosocial metaphors of physical distress among MS patients. A 37-year-old woman living with MS expresses metaphorically her fear of losing her independence and mobility by buying shoes: "Shoes and boots being the metaphor for mobility and freedom" (p. 636). I fear losing my mobility and I fear losing my sight. Last year, I bought a pair of white roller skates and I skated. I lost my balance, fell, and landed in the emergency room. I challenge myself every day by succeeding as a mother, wife, counselor, student, daughter, friend . . . and I dare not give up! I am constantly aware of my symptoms—of my sensations or lack of sensations; however, I defy the identity of being a patient and struggle with accepting the "sick" me.

My intention for writing this personal statement is to comprehend and find meaning in the experience of living with multiple sclerosis. I explore this phenomenon from the perspective of a person living with MS who was first diagnosed at the age of 33. MS has changed my life and the lives of others who live and struggle with the challenges caused by the illness. Thus, I attempt to bring some light to the phenomenon on how a person with multiple sclerosis experiences life. I seek to understand questions such as "What is it like to experience discomfort? What does it mean to make meaning of new challenges brought about by MS? What is it like to accept MS and make meaning of the situation?" I have always known that MS was a private issue and that its disclosure was a matter of acknowledging the illness—making it public to others and myself. In a course in graduate school, I made it public. I became interested as to how this experience has influenced life. Multiple sclerosis, for example, can gradually or suddenly take your independence away. There is felt humiliation as the person regresses—now you may not be able to walk, so you become rooted like a tree as you sit in a chair.

It is difficult to learn how to cope with an unpredictable disease. What works today does not work tomorrow. We experience flare-ups and we learn about the illness. It is all very unpredictable. Words such as planning, goals, and objectives do not define multiple sclerosis. Multiple sclerosis has its own agenda, leaving you with limited control. Most people with multiple sclerosis share the theme of unpredictability. But now, fortunately, the new me is stronger. The new me knows comfort and discomfort and embraces the future with dignity and courage. The new me dares to live disabled and strives to be able. I like the "me" that is able to write, read, play, and drive; the "me" that sees well, walks well, feels well. That "me" is also well liked by my family and friends. When experiencing a flare-up, however, there is a new me with numbness and visual problems crippling my dreams. Yet living with the newness has also created spiritual tension in my life. There are questions with no answers. I wonder about the Lord. I question his existence. And I struggle. In the fight against multiple sclerosis, I feel I have no weapons. Doctors say that the medications can only slow down its progression.

There are different ways of dealing with an illness. I have learned that my tendency towards hiding MS from myself and others has been detrimental in that denial keeps me from slowing down when I must. But "How can we come to trust enough to surrender to our own bodily impulses when we are sick?" (Buttorff, 1991, p. 243).

DISCUSSION QUESTIONS

1. What do you believe are some of the causes of Alina's emotional reaction to the diagnosis?
2. What specific emotional reaction do you believe has the most impact on Alina ?
3. Would you have the same reaction to a diagnosis of a serous chronic disease? What if it were your spouse who had MS?
4. How did several years of marriage and having one child make the illness more devastating for Alina?

SET 3: HOW LONG? HOW OLD?

PERSPECTIVE

For the individual and the family, the reality of a severe illness or disability may last months, years, or a lifetime. The impact can last for generations. This long-term perspective often can influence the process of making decisions and living with the consequences.

EXPLORATION

1. How long should a 10-year-old child be kept on a life support system? A 38-year-old person? A 78-year-old person?
2. What factors must be considered in making these decisions?
3. What does "forever" mean to families who are responsible for the emotional and financial well being of a family member with a severe disability?
4. How long should parents be responsible for a child?
5. How long should children be responsible for parents?
6. Should families be required to pay for medical and rehabilitation services if gains are not made?
7. Should long-term care facilities be required to keep a patient after funds are exhausted?

REFERENCES

Armstrong, C. (1991). Emotional changes following brain injury: Psychological and neurological components of depression, denial and anxiety. *Journal of Rehabilitation*, April/May/June, 15–22.

Bader, J. L., & Robbins, R. (2001). Good grief!: Helping families cope. Brochure published by Alexander Graham Bell Association for the Deaf and Hard of Hearing, Inc., Washington, D.C.

Barnard, D. (1990). Healing the damaged self: Identity, intimacy, and meaning in the lives of the chronically ill. *Perspectives in Biology and Medicine, 33*, 535–546.

Boswell, B. B., Knight, S., Hamer, M., & McChesney, J. (2001). Disability and spirituality: A reciprocal relationship with implications for the rehabilitation process. *Journal of Rehabilitation, 67*(4), 20–25.

Breakey, J. W. (1997). Body image: The inner mirror. *Journal of Prosthetics and Orthotics, 9*(3), 107–112.

Brown, J. C. (1990). Loss and grief: An overview and guided imagery intervention model. *Journal of Mental Health Counseling, 12*(4), 434–445.

Buttorff, J. (1991). The lived experience of being comforted by a nurse. *Phenomenology + Pedagogy, 2*(1), 1–17.

Campbell, A. V. (1986). *The gospel of anger.* London: SPCK.

Cohen, M. S. (1999). Families coping with childhood chronic illness: A research review. *Family Systems and Health, 17*(2), 149–163.

Cogswell, B. E. (1968). Self-socialization: Re-adjustment of paraplegics in the community. *Journal of Rehabilitation, 34*, 11–15.

Coyle, P. K., & Halper, J. (2001). *Meeting the challenge of progressive multiple sclerosis.* New York: Demos Medical Publishing.

Deaton, A. V. (1986). Denial in the aftermath of traumatic brain injury: Its manifestations, measurement, and treatment. *Rehabilitation Psychology, 31*(4), 231–240.

Duval, M. L. (1984). Psychosocial metaphors of physical distress among MS patients. *Social Science & Medicine, 19*, 635–638.

Glazer, K. M., Emery, C. F., Frid, D. J., & Banyasz, R. E. (2002). Psychological predictors of adherence and outcomes among patients in cardiac rehabilitation. *Journal of Cardiopulmonary Rehabilitation, 22*(1), 40–46.

Harry, B. (2002). Trends and issues in serving culturally diverse families of children with disabilities. *The Journal of Special Education, 36*(3), 131–138.

Kendall, E., & Buys, N. (1998). An integrated model of psychosocial adjustment following acquired disability. *Journal of Rehabilitation,* July/August/September, 16–19.

Kim-Rupaow, W. S. (2001). *An introduction to Korean culture for rehabilitation service providers.* Buffalo, NY: Center for International Rehabilitation Research Information and Exchange.

Kübler-Ross, E. (1969). *On death and dying.* New York: MacMillan & Co.

Lane, N. J., (1995). A theology of anger when living with disability. *Rehabilitation Education, 9*(2), 97–111.

Lewis, K. (1983). Grief in chronic illness and disability. *Journal of Rehabilitation,* July/Aug/Sept, 8–11.

Livneh, H. (2001). Psychosocial adaptation to chronic illness and disability: A conceptual Framework. *Rehabilitation Counseling Bulletin, 44*(3), 151–160.

Livneh, H., Martz, E., & Wilson, L. M. (2001). Denial and perceived visibility as predictors of adaptation to disability among college students. *Journal of Vocational Rehabilitation, 16*(3/4), 227–234.

Longo, D. A., & Peterson, S. M. (2002). The role of spirituality in psychosocial rehabilitation. *Psychiatric Rehabilitation Journal, 25*(4), 333–340.

Marinelli. R. P., & Dell Orto, A. E. (1999). *Psychological and social aspects of physical disability.* New York: Springer Publishing.

Martin, S. A. (1986). Anger as inner transformation. *Quadrant, 19*(1).

Martz, E. (2002). *Adaptation to disability and post-traumatic stress disorder: An empirical study on the reactive phases to the trauma of disability.* Columbia, MO: University of Missouri.

Matt, D. A., Sementilli, M. E., & Burish, T.G. (1988). Denial as a strategy for coping with cancer. *Journal of Mental Health Counseling, 10* (2), 136–144.

Miller, E. T. (2002). Targeting interventions for primary informal caregivers of adults with cognitive and physical losses. *Rehabilitation Nursing, 27*(2), 46–51.

O'Connor, R. (1997). *Undoing depression.* New York: Berkley Books.

Pearson, J. (1973). Behavioral aspects of Huntington's Chorea. *Advances in Neurology, 1*, 701–712.

Power, P. W., & Dell Orto, A. E. (1980). *Role of the family in the rehabilitation of the physically disabled.* Baltimore: University Park Press.

Power, P. W., Dell Orto, A. E., & Gibbons, M. B. (1988). *Family interventions throughout chronic illness and disability.* New York: Springer Publishing.

Rolland, J. S. (1994). *Families, illness & disability.* New York: Basic Books.

Santana, S., & Santana, O. (2001). *An introduction to Mexican culture for rehabilitation service providers. Buffalo, NY:* Center for International Rehabilitation Research Information and Exchange.

Shontz, F. C. (1978). Psychological adjustment to physical disability: Trends in theories. *Archives of Physical Medicine and Rehabilitation, 59,* 251–254.

Stanhope, V. (2002). Culture, control, and family involvement: A comparison of psychosocial rehabilitation in India and the United States. *Psychiatric Rehabilitation Journal, 25*(30), 273–280.

Watson, M., Green, S., Blake, S., & Schrapnell, K. (1984). Reaction to a diagnosis of breast cancer: Relationship between denial, delay, and rates of psychological morbidity. *Cancer, 53,* 2008–2012.

Weihs, K., Fisher, L., & Baird, M. (2002). Families, health, and behavior. *Family Systems and Health, 20*(1), 7–46.

Weisman, A. (1972). *On death and dying.* New York: Behavioral Publications.

Yoshida, K. K. (1993). Reshaping of self: A pendular reconstruction of self and identity among adults with traumatic spinal cord injury. *Sociology of Health and Illness, 15,* 217–245.

4

Family Response to Illness and Disability

The illness or disability of a family member challenges the core values and resources of the family system. Not only must the family adapt to the emerging needs of the person with the medical condition, but it must also continue to maintain a sense of unity by regrouping its members, refocusing its resources, and redefining its functions. How the family reorganizes depends upon its emotional response to the loss, stress, hope, and reality consequent to the illness or disability (Williams & Kay, 1991; Kosciulek, 1994; MacFarlene, 1999).

The family is not just affected by chronic illness or severe disability. It can positively influence the recovery and eventual adjustment process (Cohen, 1999). With the impact of a traumatic medical condition, many family members are forced into a life transition—a redefinition of family expectations and responsibilities takes place (Faulkner & Davey, 2002). Though family members may experience many changes, they still can and often must play an integral role in the wellbeing of the individual who is disabled or ill (Knox, Parmester, Atkinson, & Yazbeck, 2000).

This chapter explores how family members react to the complexities, challenges, and demands of the medical experience. Bringing these reactive patterns into sharper focus can enhance the understanding of the influences the family can have on the stabilization, treatment, and rehabilitation of the person who has the illness or disability. An explanation of these family reactions is often embedded in the identification of the determinants of these responses and the cultural expectations of a specific time period (Ferguson, 2002). To be noted, however, is that since each family is unique, changing, and evolving, so are the reactions to the life related changes of a family member. This chapter will also describe the many family needs emerging from their emotional responses, as well as the concerns reported by family members. These determinants, reactions, needs, and shared problems generate distinctive adaptive tasks for the family. All of these issues are outlined in

Tables 4.1 and 4.2. A structure for understanding family behaviors is to identify specific periods following the initial trauma. Family behaviors may vary according to a particular phase in the treatment and rehabilitation process

DETERMINANTS OF FAMILY REACTION TO ILLNESS OR DISABILITY

There are many causes for family reactions to an illness or disability. These factors may not only indicate why a family is reacting in a particular way, but also what may be done by health care professionals and other support systems to assist the family in adjusting to a complex, demanding, and changing reality (Rolland, 1994). These influences or sources are placed into the following groups: family characteristics, illness/disability related characteristics, developmental stages, and cultural/ environmental issues.

FAMILY CHARACTERISTICS

There are certain factors that are thematic to all families when understanding the sources of the family's emotional response. These include risk and protective issues, belief systems, availability of coping resources, previous history, family communication styles and interactive relationships, and who is ill or disabled in the family system.

1. **Risk factors.** Many families are vulnerable to those behaviors that impede the adjustment of the person who is ill or disabled. Such factors as lack of any adequate support systems, intrafamilial conflict, blame and criticism, unrelentless external stress, and family composition, such as a single parent or divorced spouse, can create a family situation that inhibits any resilience to the impact of a severe medical condition (Weihs, Fisher, & Baird, 2002). The illness or disability situation generates distress in other family members that is exacerbated by these risk factors, and the heightened distress prevents these persons from meeting the needs of the affected family member.

The factors of blame and guilt can be strong undercurrents for family members regardless of the cause of the injury. The perception of personal responsibility for the cause of an illness or disability can be a significant determinant in family member adaptation. If the person with a disability takes responsibility for engaging in the behavior that

TABLE 4.1   Selected Needs That Provide Guidelines for Intervention Strategies

Time Period	Determinants For all time periods	Reactions	Needs
Diagnosis/ beginning of treatment or re-habilitation	Family characteristics Illness/disability Characteristics Developmental stages Cultural/ environmental	Shock, anger, in-tense anxiety, grief, guilt Helplessness	Respect Concern Listen Support Working relation-ship with health professionals
Course of hospi-tal treatment and rehabilitation		Depression Hope Anger Denial Anxiety over the future Coping strategies	Maintain control Reassurance and hope Gain perspective Support Create meaning that promotes family com-petence
Return to avail-able family and outpatient status		Lingering guilt Hope Anxiety Coping strategies Gradual realization Reorientation	Information Manage stress Time and energy into themselves Enlarge scope of values Role redefinition and reclaim fam-ily life Gradual realization Support Maintain family boundaries

TABLE 4.2   Determinants, Reactions, and Needs, and Shared Problems Generate Distinctive Adaptive Tasks

Time Period	Adaptive Tasks
Diagnosis/beginning of	Maintain equilibrium and essential family treatment/rehabilitationfunctions
Course of hospital	Adjustment to condition/treatment/rehabilitation Utilize support systems Recognize potential family problems
Return to available family	Neutralize environmental conditions and outpatient status Maintenance of family support systems Tolerate stressors Re-orientation

caused the accident, such as alcohol consumption or not wearing a seatbelt, other family members may adapt more easily to post-injury adjustment demands. Other family members may then feel less guilty. But even with this assumption of personal responsibility, family communications may be blame-laden or used as ammunition in family power struggles.

2. **Protective factors.** Many family members, however, are capable of easily connecting with the person who is ill or disabled and providing support and attention to specific needs. Among family members there may be also a congruence of beliefs, an ability to engage in effective problem solving—to communicate directly with each other, to find time for recreational activities, and to establish satisfying relationship with health providers (Weihs, Fisher, & Baird, 2002). All of these factors help family members regulate the distress engendered by the medical event.

3. **Belief systems.** How the family organizes itself to manage illness or disability-related demands, their understanding of causes of family life changes during treatment and rehabilitation, and how they connect with health care providers is often a reflection of a family belief system. In turn, this system is influenced by cultural and religious values (Rolland, 1994). Further, the communication of appropriate information by health professionals concerning care-giving responsibilities can have a decided impact on family beliefs. Early communication of appropriate knowledge of illness and disability-related issues may also change the family's understanding of the illness or disability. Yet understanding

does not mean there is a positive outcome. A change in understanding can create higher expectations for the eventual adjustment of the family member. If the family is in doubt about the illness/disability implications for the injured family member, this uncertainty will create continued family tension and inhibit the formulation of realistic goals.

4. **Availability of coping resources.** Coping behaviors represent one expression of how family members respond to an unexpected change in family life caused by illness/disability, and for these behaviors to be initiated demands personal and environmental resources. Personality strengths that have been honed and developed by life experience, such as an optimistic attitude, a persistent style that is accustomed to confronting new challenges, and the learned ability to utilize available support opportunities, can all facilitate positive coping behaviors. These available resources may include personal values grounded in religious beliefs or expectations from influential others that firmly suggest that changes related to a disability or illness can be dealt with realistically. Also, other coping resources include existing and satisfying work activity, support from extended family, availability of necessary community resources, anticipation of planned activities, and self-help groups which can be helpful in times of the continued stress associated with the illness or disability experience. Included in these resources are financial means and the ability of family members to use community agencies. A family that has financial protection will theoretically cope much better than one for whom illness or disability represents a financial disaster. However, some financially secure families have become emotionally bankrupt while poorer families have not only survived but also have become emotionally rich. Given the astronomical costs associated with health care, few families can feel that they are completely secure from the long-term financial issues related to lifetime care.

5. **Previous family history.** Family history includes the mental and physical health of the family members, as well as how the family has dealt with previous crises (Rolland, 1994). A chronic physical or emotional illness may seriously hamper the expression of energy required for most care-giving efforts. If a family member has a past history of mental illness, the family experience of living with the added adjustment demands of a physical disability may only trigger memories of painful and unpleasant times, even though the mental illness is now managed. Also, when a life crisis is an unfamiliar event, the family will usually display confusion and have a more difficult time focusing its resources. When previous crises have identified family resources and helped to establish coping patterns, then the impact of the disability may be less devastating. Shock and a feeling of helplessness will still be present

after the initial diagnosis, but these reactions may be managed more readily if the family has successfully managed other losses. A family whose breadwinner has been out of work for many months because of an illness or disability, for example, has often had an opportunity to assess its resources as well as expand them. If another member of the family is diagnosed with a severe illness a few years later, the family may have the ability to adapt successfully if its resources were used effectively during the previous illness. If coping patterns have been effective in the past, then they will usually be adopted again in the new crisis. However, past success should be considered in the context of the families' inability to deal with the adjustment demands prompted by a new stressor, such as a debilitating chronic illness, because their resources have not been replenished and new skills have not been developed relevant to the unique aspects of the disability.

6.   **Family communication styles and interactive relationships.** A family system that is nurturing, well-structured, and has a communication style that represents openness, a freedom to express feelings without fear of criticism, and a listening ear from others has the potential for an adaptive response to the transitions caused by the illness/disability. In contrast, members of a family who are indecisive, have contradictory types of behavior, and possess a communication pattern characterized more by blame and criticism, will generally act in isolation from one another and have a difficult time reaching out for mutual support. The illness or disability experience for this family will usually bring protracted periods of confusion and avoidance behavior when confronting the realistic implications of the serious medical event.

7.   **Who is ill or disabled in the family system.** A differential response among family members may be caused by whether it is a child, adolescent, parent, or spouse who becomes chronically ill or severely disabled. Attachments, hopes, dreams, and expectations are all issues surrounding the losses emerging from a sudden change in one of the family members. A severe disability of a husband and father, however, who is regarded by family members as the primary breadwinner but who undergoes a radical change in employment status may have a lasting effect on the quality and status of family life. Future plans involving education and upward mobility may have to be significantly altered.

A child who becomes severely disabled resulting from an accident will, of course, precipitate shock and intense feelings of sadness and anxiety. The illness or disability of a child can be frequently regarded as "off-time," facilitating a chronic sorrow accompanying family living. Any severe medical condition in any family member usually causes intense sadness, but this condition affecting a child may bring its own distinctive array of emotions. Also, a child's disability can easily result in intense stress if the parents are unable to help each other during the acute stage of adjustment.

DISABILITY OR ILLNESS-RELATED CHARACTERISTICS

The visibility of a disability, the uncertainty of the illness outcome, the problematic and unpredictable course of a disease, and how the nature of the disability affects family functioning are all determinants of the family's response (Chan, 2000). Some neurological disorders, for example, cause awkward body movements or spontaneous verbal outbursts, e.g., Huntington's disease. Other diseases such as AIDS and specific forms of mental illness often are the subject of stigma. All of these diagnoses can create embarrassment, isolation, fear, and intense anxiety among family members. Also, if several physical accommodations have to be constructed in the home, such modifications may be viewed as disruptions in customary patterns of family life and, in turn, may generate anger and resentment. Moreover, if a chronic illness is inherited, younger family members may live in constant anxiety because of uncertainty over whether they will be affected. Further, an illness and its accompanying care-giving responsibilities that extend over a long period of time may eventually become emotionally draining for certain family members, leaving them in a state of exhaustion and vulnerable to depression.

DEVELOPMENTAL STAGES

Each family stage brings the necessity of accomplishing certain tasks, i.e., raising children or building financial security for the family. The presence of a disability or chronic illness can have a unique impact on the family if the children have left home and the parents have been planning for their retirement years. Suddenly they are aware of diminished, available support systems and may be looking at nursing homes or coma management facilities rather than retirement homes.

A developmental stage that occurs in the later years of a family's history does not mean that the occurrence of a disability or chronic illness is "on time." Severe medical traumas are never "on time," though many family members as they mature may realize that a disability or chronic illness is not totally unexpected. This sense that an unwelcome medical event "could happen" may cushion the emotional impact of the diagnosis. The initial responses of shock and resentment may fortunately not linger and are replaced by coping strategies that attend to organizing one's resources to deal with the problem. But a gnawing disappointment and persistent feelings of loss may exist as a cloud over the remaining years of a shared family life.

Environmental/Cultural Issues

The environmental context in which a family lives includes many components such as available support systems, positive or negative attitudes from health professionals and other professionals who interact with the family, varied community resources, e.g., neighbors or community organizations, extended family members, and family friendly employers and schools (Muscott, 2002). Support systems are defined as continuing social aggregates (namely, continuing interactions with another individual, network, group, or organization), which provide individuals with opportunities for feedback about themselves and validation of their expectations of others (Caplan, 1976). The availability of an extended family, support group, or similar resource can make a difference in how a family copes with a disability experience (Curtiss, Klemz, & Vanderploeg, 2000; Lin, 2000). These resources may provide respite care, nurturance, and feelings of acceptance to the family that conveys the message that despite what has happened each family member is a worthwhile human being.

Most families are embedded in a context of cultural diversity, which negates the possibility of only viewing cultural realities as simply traditional or even discrete influences (Harry, 2002). The family's culture makes a decided difference in the member's adjustment to the disability (Hampton & Marshall, 2000; Santana & Santana, 2001). The attributions for disability and illness, the value attached to the condition, and the extent of stigma differ widely among and within ethnic groups (Harry, 2002). The acculturation process also has a significant impact on caregiving styles.

African-American families, for example, are organized around extended kinship networks that may include blood and nonrelated persons (Rogers-Dulon & Blacher, 1995). Family roles, responsibilities, and functions are often interchanged among family members, a sharing which cuts across generations and gender roles (Carter & Cook, 1991; Cavallo & Savcedo, 1995). There is variability among Latin American families (e.g., Puerto Rican, Cuban, and Mexican) with regard to ethnicity and class differences (Santana & Santana, 2001). Traditional

Latino cultural values of fatalism, respect, spirituality, and personalism may often be reflected in their adjustment to a disability event (Dillard, 1983). Within Asian families, moreover, transgenerational beliefs on coping with illness can be particularly important (Hampton & Marshall, 2000). The concept of obligation is also central in Asian cultures and families, and family obligations such as providing care for a disabled family member are indirectly communicated using nonconfrontational strategies (Carter & Cook, 1991). In other words, all families have distinctive cultural values and the impact of these values on the characteristics of disability and/or illness adjustment play a significant part in a families' reactive pattern to disability and illness.

The different determinants, consequently, can suggest and accurately identify why family members are showing specific behaviors as they respond to a chronic illness or disability. Added to family beliefs, which Rolland (1994) has identified as key variables influencing the family's response to an illness or disability, are two other determinants that he believes contribute to disability's impact on the family. They are the family's multigenerational, evolutionary process with illness, loss, and crisis, and the family's sense of mastery and control over the course of an illness. They are actually components of family beliefs, and further suggest whether the family can become a valuable resource or support system during the family member's treatment and rehabilitation process.

Importantly, each family is unique in the way it reacts to a medical situation, and often there are several causes to an individual family member's reaction. Anger, for example, may be prompted both by unfinished business that exists within a family over unresolved grievances and by a stage in the family life cycle when a married couple are embarking on their own life without the immediate responsibility of children. Suddenly a young adult becomes severely disabled, canceling future plans for the parents. But among all the identified determinants, two pivotal considerations to understanding any influence on family emotional responses are to pinpoint who is ill or disabled in the family system and the changes that are therefore necessary in family life because of the medical situation, and what is the nature of the illness or disability. A disease that has an indefinite course of treatment may stimulate many emotions such as confusion, intense anxiety, depression, and an endless search for a meaning to the medical event.

FAMILY REACTION TO CHRONIC ILLNESS

Historically, there have been many contributions from researchers on family reactive patterns to long-term illness (Bray, 1977; Epperson, 1977;

Faulkner & Davey, 2002; Ferguson, 2002; Weihs, Fisher, & Baird, 2002; Giaquinta, 1977; Livneh, 2001). These models or concepts are usually more appropriate when there are clear phases or steps in illness or disability progression and when the end result is more or less predictable. Armstrong (1991) believes, for example, that family reactions to traumatic brain injury, for example, are likely to follow a developmental course, beginning with a response to acute stress that is reactive and crisis-oriented.

The identification of information of family responses provides further knowledge about which responses encourage the family's ability to cope and which do not. Families develop effective ways to deal with the illness or disability situation when they attempt to normalize family life and change appropriately their own individual role expectations to deal with family demands. But if individual family members harbor their own grief, guilt, and anger, and project these emotions in a negative manner onto each other and health professionals, or deny the important family implications of the diagnosis such as necessary role reallocations and changes in many family routines, then the family may never adjust to the disability experience. A lingering resistance to acknowledging one's role in working toward family adjustment may also precipitate nonfacilitative coping responses (Dell Orto & Power, 1994).

There are many considerations that provide a foundation upon which to build an understanding of the dynamics of a family's reaction to disability and illness. When conceptualizing a family's illness reaction, a number of authors have proposed stages of coping, especially when a child's disability is diagnosed. These stages are an adaptation of Kübler-Ross' (1969) stages of grief experienced after the death of a loved one (Muscott, 2002). However, the phases of grief related to the course of an illness after the diagnosis typically include some variations of shock, emotional disorganization, and emotional adjustment (Blacher, 1984). Since there are varied reactions from family members, this variation limits the generalization of stage theories to understanding how other families are dealing with even a similar trauma.

Any perspective on family reactions to illness and disability should convey the reality that families are usually confronted with constraints against using specific coping resources or experiencing positive emotions leading to effective disability and family management. These constraints may be personal, such as internalized cultural values and beliefs that proscribe certain types of action or feelings, and personal agendas (e.g., fear of failure or unfinished business), or environmental issues (e.g., lack of available resources or negative, stereotypic attitudes from health professionals) (Power, 1995).

It is important to note that, family reactive models have undergone an evolution since 1965. Focusing primarily on reactive patterns to child disability, initially the research reflected the belief that parents were dysfunctional, and family responses were determined by a "damaged family" (Ferguson, 2002). Later, parents were viewed more as "suffering" and the interplay of parental emotions with the environmental circumstances was emphasized. Anger, guilt, and denial were replaced by loneliness, stress, and chronic sorrow. But since 1980 an adaptational perspective has emerged, influenced by disability-related legislation and family support programs (Ferguson, 2002). Attention is now given to those reactive factors that encourage family resilience and adaptation, particularly taking into account that family members vary tremendously in how they respond to the same event in their lives.

Another way to conceptualize the family's reactions to a trauma is to identify different emotions and coping mechanisms expressed by family members that may occur not in stages but at any time during the family member's treatment and rehabilitation. These emotions and coping styles may subside and then recur unexpectedly. They are dynamic processes that may emerge, continue, and then wane in the course of time. Many recurrent emotions are also manifestations of individual coping styles such as anger and loss of hope.

There is yet another approach to understanding the reactions of family members to illness and disability. The extensive range of negative phenomena associated with caring for persons has been called "caregiver burden" (Chwallisz, 1992). The amount of burden a family member experiences can depend on age, gender, coping styles, how one views the situation, and mental health history prior to the trauma. Objective burden is understood as problems encountered by the person, such as environmental changes experienced by the caregiver, i.e., financial strain, change of role, or employment status (Allen, Linn, Gutierrez, & Willer, 1994). Subjective burden is perceived stress, or the amount of psychological strain on family members that is caused by changes in the person with head trauma. Perceived stress, however, is difficult to define precisely. What may be appraised as harmful or threatening to one family member may not be considered as challenging to another. However, personal burdens are realities caused by daily management responsibilities, perceived limits on family opportunities, and perhaps the lack of personal rewards that persons may experience when caring for the injured.

Unfortunately, all of the family reactive models do not provide any information on why some families mange to adapt while others become entrenched in a posture of resistance to change (Rape, Bush, & Slavin, 1992). If the family is viewed as a constantly interactive group of unique individuals, family members will exhibit differential adaptation patterns following the trauma. Also, a specific response may be more applicable to one family member than another.

When identifying family reactions to an illness or disability, frequently the emotional responses of siblings are overlooked. But children of a parent who is experiencing a severe medical condition, or siblings of a child who has a chronic illness or severe disability, have distinctive responses which can either facilitate or hinder the family's eventual adaptation. Though the reaction will vary according to his or her developmental stages, each young person will be affected by the trauma. In some instances the adolescent may become the parent (Keydel, 1988). The nature of the illness may also affect the response. Faulkner and Davey (2000) reported from their study that mothers diagnosed with breast cancer discovered that their adolescent daughters became resentful, more argumentative, and emotionally and physically distanced themselves from the ill parent. Overall, the daughters had more difficulty coping with their mother's condition than the sons.

Inherited illnesses may prompt the response among siblings, "Am I going to get what my sister or brother has?" Anxiety is heightened among the children in a family whose parents are severely disabled, or they may attempt to deny the trauma by not discussing it at all. Siblings who are well may feel depressed or unworthy, unable to tolerate the unfairness of being whole and healthy while their sibling is living with the medical condition (Palmer, Kriegsman, & Palmer, 2000). Sadness, irritability, academic difficulties, and fears are added emotions and behaviors experienced by children affected by a parental disability or illness (Urbach, Sonenklar, & Culbart, 1994). But many children in a similar family situation cope quite well and become resources of strength and hope for adult family members. They frequently take the initiative in building social support networks with peers and other family members, modify their recreational arrangements to accommodate parental limitations, and willingly assist in many care-giving functions (Blackford, 1999).

Though within one family its members may display varied responses to the medical event, many of these reactions could be characterized as dysfunctional. If family members perceive that dealing with caregiving responsibilities is beyond their ability, or view the illness or disability as either a disaster or unfair, then they might see themselves as victims. Blaming each other for the trauma, denying the reality of what has occurred, showing no tolerance for other family members, and refusing to display necessary role flexibility are examples of poor coping responses and behaviors. On the other hand, perspectives that include optimism, faith, and courage, and maintaining open and clear commu-

nication among members can be helpful to families as they attempt to
the changes in family life.

A further approach to understanding a family's response to disability
is in the context of definite time frames occurring from onset of the
trauma throughout the course of treatment and rehabilitation. These
time frames, identified in Table 4.1, are diagnosis/beginning of treatment or rehabilitation, the course of hospital treatment and rehabilitation, and return to the available family and outpatient status. Each
frame can be called a "trigger" point, a period in which family members
may be especially vulnerable to excessive stress and a time when a series
of tasks may have to be negotiated by them (Caroff & Mailick, 1985;
Power, 1991). During these time periods, moreover, different emotional
responses can emerge, subside, and re-emerge during the course of an
illness of disability. The emotions can be conceptualized as reactive
themes, and are explained below:

THEMES

Shock

The onset of a chronic illness or disability has a sudden, unexpected,
and usually extensive effect on the life of family members. Feelings of
helplessness, numbness, being overwhelmed, confusion, and perhaps
even the temporary loss of self-control result from the initial event. At
this time family members need to feel they have hope and that hospital
personnel care about the patient.

Denial

With little information or understanding as to what extent the person
will be impaired or of illness outcome, family members may deny any
implications of the trauma regarding permanent physical, emotional,
or intellectual limitations. Denial may also take the form of insistence
that the recovery be complete, divine intervention will occur, and minimal future changes to family life will occur. At this time, the denial
may serve a positive purpose. Entertaining hopes may give family members the time and opportunity to identify and organize their coping
resources.

Grief

Grief is a persistent feeling in families, an emotion resulting not only
from the realities of family disruption, but also from the loss of a

family partner with whom family members had a mutual and caring relationship (Bader & Robbins, 2001). All of a sudden it becomes a one-way relationship and they miss the person who cared about them in a special way (Mitiguy, 1990). In fact, grief may be especially poignant for the injured person's spouse since the essential loss of a partner is mourned. This mourning is borne alone because society neither recognizes the grief nor provides the support and comfort that usually surrounds those bereaved (Zeigler, 1987). Depending on the nature of the disability or illness, grief may continue because family members remain in an uncertain state; they're waiting for full recovery, but realize that they may be dealing with the patient's impairments for the rest of their lives.

COPING STRATEGIES

Integral to understanding the manner in which families react to the brain injury situation is the awareness that family members will utilize different coping mechanisms as they attempt to adjust to living with the injury (Orsillo, McCaffrey, & Fisher, 1993). Certain varied coping strategies may be used for a period of time only to then be replaced by other mechanisms. Coping strategies are employed to manage stressful demands, ward off threats to family life, and perhaps even to change the situation. Families who appear to adapt well utilize, with other resources, a more cognitive style of coping that expresses a sense of mastery in regard to their circumstances. Mastery can comprise a variety of skills, assigning positive meaning to the difficulties associated with family changes and pinpointing the personal reasons why one is responding negatively to these family disruptions.

Cognitive coping styles may also embrace beliefs that influence family adjustment (Lustig, 2002). These beliefs include (a) a shared commitment and purpose, (b) framing life and events as more optimistic and beneficial, (c) feeling more tolerant and less judgmental, and (d) developing an ability to live successfully with the unknown course of treatment or the eventual outcome (Bramlett, Hall, Barnett, & Rowell, 1995; Scorgie, Wilgosh, & McDonald, 1996). Muscott (2002) also reports that Olson and colleagues (1983) have identified five categories of coping styles that families use to deal with stress: (a) passive appraisal, (b) reframing, (c) spiritual support, (d) social support, and (e) professional support. Family members may rely more heavily at certain times on one form of coping, for example, defensive strategies, and at other times on other forms, such as problem-solving strategies. Examples of problem-solving strategies are information seeking, taking direct action, turning to others for help, and tension reduction techniques.

Pearlin and Schooler (1978) have suggested the following three categories that are very relevant to illness and disability.

1.   Strategies to change the family situation (stress, anxiety, confusion, and avoidance by family members), caused by illness or disability. These can include seeking advice and information from knowledgeable persons, and tapping one's own individual strengths, such as communication skills and ability to identify valuable community resources.

2.   Strategies to control, not change, family disruptions, anxieties, uncertainties for the future, and feelings of grief and loss. These strategies include positive comparisons formulated by family members ("We could be worse off . . . "), entertaining beliefs that the patient will improve somewhat or that support for care-giving responsibilities is available, utilizing tension reduction approaches, such as relaxation training or pursuing recreational activities, and accumulating knowledge.

3.   Strategies to minimize personal discomforts caused by the reality of disability, such as stress, fear, frustration, disappointment, and future uncertainties. These strategies include venting (talking with others about one's problems), distracting oneself with activities, stoically accepting the situation, and even wishful thinking, namely, imagining that someday the family situation will be better. For many family members' prayers can also be an invaluable help to minimize feelings of grief and loss.

The coping strategies used by family members will generally depend on how the individual family member appraises the situation of living with the illness/disability experience and his or her perception of the resources available. An individual makes a series of judgments concerning the potential effects of events on their emotional well being. In other words, coping involves not only behavior, but also varied thoughts on how best to deal with the situation.

FAMILY NEEDS

Emerging from the varied family emotional reactions are selected needs that provide guidelines for intervention strategies and are identified in Table 4.1. These needs will frequently differ according to the time period of the family member's course of treatment and rehabilitation

(Stebbins & Leung, 1998). Some of these needs will be constant through-out the entire period of illness or disability progression. The importance of possessing appropriate information, seeking support, interacting with health professionals, and recognizing potential problems are usually thematic to all time periods after the initial medical trauma. At appro-priate times, family members need their questions answered honestly and explanations given in understandable terms (Mathis, 1984). Sup-port, however, may take different forms during the different time peri-ods. Initially, support to a family may be expressed by providing a listening ear to their own fears and uncertainties about the perceived family losses. Later, support may be given by identifying community resources, including those offering financial assistance. Frequently fam-ily members are not aware of their own needs, and other family members or health professionals could identify them (Kolakowsky-Hayner, Miner, & Kreutzer, 2001).

FAMILY ADAPTIVE TASKS

With the family's slow acknowledgment that the effects of the disability will be permanent, individual family members will gradually adjust their life to meet care-giving demands, role reallocation tasks, and perhaps family finance changes. Reorientation is both a continuous, adaptive process and a necessary task for family adjustment. It represents the achievement of selected goals during the family's long adjustment pe-riod. Developmental changes in young persons or changes in the differ-ent phases of marital life may influence a shift in family duties and roles. The worsening of an illness or disability condition may also cause major family changes.

Although grieving can take on a chronic nature, many families do eventually work through feelings of denial, optimism, anger, and depres-sion to a degree of adjustment (Lustig, 1999). For some, this can take several years with varying amounts of time for family members to come to some sense of resolution and acceptance. Yet many families start to educate themselves, seek out supports, assess problems, and plan for the future (Waaland & Kreutzer, 1988). During this period of reorientation, fears about the patient's present and future preoccupy the stressed relatives (Armstrong, 1991; Kreutzer, Devany, & Bergquist, 1994).

This reorientation of personal lives within the context of family life is usually very difficult for family members. Feelings of blame, anger, and resentment still linger, even accompanied by both a sense of relief that the injured person did survive and a conviction of hope that previous functions will return.

During this time of reorientation, however, as the injured person is slowly reintegrated into family life, the family should undertake specific tasks. These tasks are in harmony with the emotional responses and consequent needs of all family members and actually identify intervention goals. These tasks could be thematic to the different time periods involved in family adaptation to illness and disability, and are identified in Table 4.2.

1. *Maintain family equilibrium.* Gradually, a balance should be established between the necessary changes in family life and the continuation and stability of necessary family roles. Often such equilibrium is not attained until the family member who is ill or disabled returns to the family home and care-giving responsibilities go into effect. Information, support, and family member flexibility are key factors in developing this balance.

2. *Utilize support systems.* Frequently, family members have to arrive at a time in their own reaction to the medical trauma that they believe they are either ready to reach out for some form of assistance from others, or are open to the initiating efforts of others to provide some kind of help. Family members who are still in a state of complete denial about what has occurred, or who are intensely angry and resentful about the loss, may not be disposed to receive necessary support at that time. The utilization of effective support demands timing.

3. *Recognize potential family problems.* Such recognition is both a need and a task. Different family concerns will surface during the entire course of treatment and rehabilitation, and the awareness and appraisal that a concern could become a difficult problem may be a beginning to maintaining an acceptable quality of family life. The awareness presumes that there are open communication patterns among family members.

4. *Tolerate stressors.* Tolerance for the many personal and family changes occurring during illness or disability demands many different interventions. Tolerance can be wedded to effective coping, and skillful management of perceived stressors necessitates personal resources, the availability of support systems, appropriate information, and positive relationships with health professionals.

As the family engages in their adaptive tasks, and in their understanding that both anger and depression are parts of the grieving process, the physical, personal, social, familial, vocational, and economic ramifications of the disability become apparent. Some families may welcome these changes and perceive living with the disability as a means for renewed family togetherness. Other families may view the necessary changes as manageable and they may believe that their adjustment to the disability is an expression of their commitment and endurance, perceiving the family future as unalterably shaped. Still other families may perceive that the changes caused by an injury are catastrophic (Kreutzer, Devany, & Bergquist, 1994). They feel the future of the person with the disability is hopeless, and that family life will now be characterized as troubled and lonely.

Unique to each family, and influenced by their cultural heritage, are other possible adaptive tasks, such as quickly gaining a sense of competence in handling family affairs after a sudden disruption in family life, becoming more assertive in order to deal effectively with health professionals, and providing support to a family decision maker who, because of cultural reasons, assumes primary responsibility for keeping the family together. But adaptation to a severe illness or disability event is ongoing, and the family's long-term adjustment might be considerably altered as their perceptions of living with the disability change (Keydel, 1991). All of the adaptive tasks, however, connect with planned, family interventions to achieve the reality that a family is attempting to do the best it can under difficult circumstances.

CONCLUSION

There is an increasing body of reported research that suggests that most families do adapt satisfactorily to a chronic illness or disability (Ferguson, 2002). Especially for families associated with raising a child with disabilities, a significant number of parents report many benefits and positive outcomes. The question still lingers, however, "Why are some families more resilient than others when faced with a severe medical trauma?" The answer is as varied as are the families affected by the condition. What helps when exploring a satisfactory answer is the identification and understanding of how family members are responding to what has happened. An appraisal of their reactions opens the door for acknowledging the needs and problem areas related to the illness/disability occurrence. All of this knowledge establishes the foundation for successful family interventions.

TED AND HIS MOTHER: HOW LIFE SUDDENLY CHANGES

As this chapter indicates, there are varied reactions among family members to the personal experience of a severe disability or a chronic illness.

The causes of the medical event often determine the type of individual and family response. Such reactions are also cyclic, and can also be influenced by who is available to provide support. The following account describes a multitude of reactions by both a son and his mother, and identifies how specific circumstances and available people can make a difference in how one reacts to a medical situation from disability onset through treatment and eventual rehabilitation.

Son: Changing from a fully functioning, young, athletic college student to a comatose, nonverbal invalid can take place in a matter of seconds. To recover may require years; some may never recover. For me, being alive today is a miracle. Following the motorcycle accident that resulted in a brain stem contusion, my family was informed that it was unlikely that I would live. The following presentation is a perspective on our personal struggle to beat the odds from my standpoint and that of my mother. Not only were we able to win, we were also able to rise above the physical and emotional strain placed on our lives.

As a college student, I was at the point in my life of having everything going for me. I was happy as a student at a northeastern United States university, had a girlfriend, and was actively involved as a member of the track team. My preoccupations at that time centered around my independence, my future, and the variety of other joys and pleasures which were part of my life and that of my friends. The summer prior to my senior year I was employed as a construction worker. To reduce the amount of time I would have to spend traveling to my home, I was living in a tent. It was a taste of the pioneer life, living in the outdoors, working, and basically enjoying my sense of independence from my family. This need for independence and self-sufficiency had been an issue in the relationship with my parents and had caused some conflict between us. At this time I had no idea that I would soon become the most helpless, dependent person imaginable.

One day before my senior year, I was riding my motorcycle, enjoying the beauty of the summer evening. My last recollection was that I was out of control. The next thing I remembered was that it was November and I was in a hospital. Since I had no speech and was partially paralyzed, my life at that time was one of confusion, desperation, and challenge. I had a hard time putting the pieces together, but I somehow realized that I was hurting. I know that I needed people to maintain my life supports since I could not do anything on my own. My decision at that time was that if I was going to survive, I must draw people to me. I could not act up because I might drive them away.

Mother: The call from a doctor in the accident room of the medical center reported that my son's condition was "grave" and that he had stopped breathing several times. I felt very calm as I reminded the doctor that he had been an associate of my late father and that I wished everything to be done for my son. He was in the critical care section, convulsing and surrounded by aides, doctors, nurses, tubes, a machine, wires —and he was dirty. My husband was sure he would live; I was sure that he would die.

The rest of the night was unreal. We learned as much as we could about the accident, then we called our daughter, relatives, and physicians, signed papers, listened to reports that gave our son a 5% chance to live. Most terrible of all was that there was nothing I could do but wait helplessly. For a month of coma, I waited. Through several infections, operations, and x-rays, I waited. I asked, "Why?" but there was no answer. I was terrified, and still there was so very little I could actively do. School began, and I returned to work. This was a very great help to me because my mind was taken up and I was active. We all experienced a sort of "yo-yo" condition—way up with hope one day, down with despair on the next. Friends, students, acquaintances, and relatives were extremely supportive. Finally, my son came out of the coma . His eyes opened, he moved, not much but a little. He would blink twice for "no" and once for "yes." I really think I had hoped it would be like a soap opera—he would open his eyes and say, "Where am I?" and get up out of bed and come home. If I had ever known how very long it would be! He was moved from the CCU to the neurological section of the hospital. This was somewhat traumatic for us all because the care was not so careful or so intensive. About this point I really came to grips with the problem. I had stopped my "whys" and self-pity, swallowed some of my overweening pride, and accepted the fact that whatever happened, God's will, and not mine, would prevail. At last I could cope.

Son: Being unable to speak since I came out of my coma, I was in a position of having to deal internally with the many issues that I was terrified and uncertain of, such as "Will I ever be able to speak, walk, or even approximate a seminormal life?" This is where the encouragement and input from the medical staff really made a difference for me. They conveyed a feeling of confidence and support that made me want to try even though I did not know how far I would be able to go. At this point in time, the personal relationships I had were just as important to me emotionally as the life supports were to me physically.

There was a critical turning point in my attitude when I began to attain some degree of independence. I became angry. I could not verbalize this anger, but it was there. It began to consume me. I went though the range of emotions, such as bitterness, hatred, disappointment, and fear. Here I was, 21 years old, a practical vegetable. How can I go on? I had a choice again: either rise above it or die emotionally, physically, or both. I chose to live, to figuratively reach out and grasp whatever bit of life I could. I attribute this choice primarily to my experience as a member of the track team and having to be independent and reach inside myself to tap resources I did not think were there—to go the extra mile. However, having made the choice, I had to still have the external motivation to go on. My nurses provided that. They were realistic, nonpatronizing, attentive to me, and made me work hard. I saw them in the same light as a coach who was there primarily to help me win. At the same time, they gave me constant input. Being unable to verbalize, I was in need of the monitoring from the outside world. It is terrifying to think what would have happened to me if I had been ignored.

Mother: Daily visits were the rule. He still could not speak, but we discovered that he could read. Physical therapy was started; he could sit up with help. He looked awful—retarded and painfully thin like a survivor of Bergen-Belsen. Our physicians were optimistic and had stopped repeating "The condition is stable; he's holding his own; his vital signs are good." How I hate those words! Tubes were removed one at a time and food, real food, was given. I was amused because our son ate everything. He'd always been an exceedingly fussy eater, and I used to threaten, "Someday you'll be so hungry, you'll eat that!" Vindication #1!

On Thanksgiving Day he came home to dinner. He still couldn't speak, had to be tied into the wheelchair so he'd not fall out, had a suprapubic catheter, and he had to be fed. But he could smile; he could communicate (sort of); and oh, how he could eat! More chicken soup? From that point on, he came home each Sunday and by Christmas he could talk, not always intelligibly, but talk. Astonishing to us all was our son's personality change. He was cheerful, cooperative, and happy (this was very different from the sometimes surly, self-conscious, and somewhat withdrawn person we were used to). Somewhere along the line he's learned to laugh at himself and to know he had to accept our help. Vindication #2! I'd told him that, too!

In February, our son was allowed to come home for a week. I was very apprehensive about this. He was pretty helpless—still had a catheter, was not very mobile, had to be dressed, etc. The one thing I'd never wanted to be was a nurse. I resent sick people, and mechanically (with tubes and such), I'm a klutz. However, I buoyed my sagging confidence by figuring I was as smart as some of the aides who'd been caring for him at the hospital (pride again). We both survived the experience. Ministering to a six-foot, two-inch baby is different. It was very difficult to return him to the hospital. But in another month he was home for good. We tried to keep everything as normal as possible. The only physical changes in the house were removing thresholds and one rug, and rearranging furniture for easier passage of the wheelchair. Again fortune smiled and sent us a young man who stayed with Ted two days of our working week, a girl who stayed one day and our housekeeper the other two. These individuals were all involved in the rehab process and were inventive therapists. I worried and tried to stave off any pitfalls. (I am still too protective.) Hospital therapy was continued on an outpatient basis, and our son worked very hard to recover. We all did.

Son: I often wonder how many severely injured or ill people live in isolation and become stagnant because they are nonresponsive like I was. This is the thought I carry with me to this day: "How lucky I was that people did care." During my hospitalization my brothers from the fraternity maintained a constant vigil. Their presence was an additional support to the family and medical personnel, especially during the difficult times when I was faced with major choices such as "Why try or why struggle?" As time passed, my attitudes of hopelessness, hatred, anger, and self-pity began to give way to hope and optimism. In retrospect, I believe this can be attributed to the small gains that I was able to make. I could feel, begin to speak, and regained a variety of body controls. While great gains were not made, there was significant progress to have me appreciate the fact that I was moving, no matter how slowly.

A traumatizing thought for me was how could I have coped if I had to remain a semiconscious vegetable for the rest of my life. When I considered the potential realities of what could have happened, I suddenly become most appreciative. As I reflect upon where I have been and where I am today, such as being able to walk, talk with a slight impediment, and remember most things, I find myself aspiring to qualitative improvement in my life. I wish that my speech could continue to improve and that I could walk better, although if I had my choice, I would choose speaking clearer over walking better.

Mother: I liked especially the honesty, humor, and realistic approach that everyone seemed to have. Questions were always answered; my only problem was in knowing what questions to ask. Our daughter took over at this point. She was preparing for two degrees, one in psychology and one in nursing. She knew what to question. Her sense of the ridiculous also smoothed some rough seas. When her brother started to talk (croak?), she spent the afternoon telling him jokes about people with speech impediments. He loved it! Whenever there was a new problem, she found the book where we could study and learn.

His physical progress was progressing. I hoped to keep his mind active and pushed him to plan to return to school. I shuddered when he could not do things that seem so easy to us who have no physical handicaps, but I tried to be less fearful for him. We took him to restaurants, to stores, and to sporting events so that he'd be used to society. He moved from the wheelchair to crutches and, oh joy!, in August he participated as an attendant in a friend's wedding. Everyone was ecstatic. He returned to college, commuting for the first semester and living at his fraternity house the second. He finally graduated. Out of 1,600 black-clad seniors, he was the one with one crutch. Now he walked, talked understandably, had a part-time job, and was accepted to graduate school. It was difficult for me to let him start off to the unfamiliar "big city" with so many problems. But I felt that he had to be independent and live his own life. He does.

Son: Interpersonally I have many friends, but I am missing one important dimension and that is a girlfriend. Prior to the accident I had a girlfriend; after it, I did not. At this time my major stumbling block is myself. I cannot see what any girl would see in me. Deep inside I guess I am hoping that I will make more gains prior to seeking out a relationship. My rationale is that the more improved I am, the better chance I have of not being rejected. However, I am aware enough to realize that the gains I make may not be tremendous and that I have to accept myself the way I am before another person could accept me. What I have going for me is my ability to place myself in situations where I can learn and experience new things. This is part of my personal rehabilitation effort to maximize my chances for success. I do not know how far I can go but I know that I will try.

Mother: How do I feel now? I have intense pride in his achievements and his hard work. I am greatly indebted to so many people for their interest and support. Most of all I'm grateful that he has been able to recover and that we as a family—my husband, my daughter, and I—have had the resources to help him. I hurt when he falls, but I try to accept it. We all try to be as realistic as possible about the future, and to face it all with gratitude, with faith, and with humor. When people ask me, and they do, how does one survive a period such as this, I quote Pearl Buck who had one of her suffering characters reply, "I really cannot face it, but I must."

DISCUSSION QUESTIONS

1. What do you believe were the causes of the varied, emotional reactions of the son during his course of treatment and rehabilitation? Did the reactions as well as behaviors change during treatment?
2. What do you believe were the causes of the mother's emotional reaction to her son's medical situation? What factors contributed to her stated "peace of mind" after many months of treatment?
3. If you became severely disabled and had to face a long period of treatment and rehabilitation, who could you rely on within your family and friends to provide the support that was evident from the son's mother?

SET 4: MY FAMILY: WHERE DO WE STAND?

Families have different ways to respond to a medical trauma of their family member. It is a difficult transition for the family and the quality of the illness/disability related family changes are determined by many factors. This structured experiential exercise helps readers to explore their own beliefs and emotions during this type of family transition.

1. List five ways your family could contribute to the care of a family member with a serious illness or disability.
2. If you were ill or disabled, would you want your family involved in your care? Why or why not?
3. What would be the most difficult aspect of family involvement for you?
5. List the characteristics of your family that help in the care of a loved one.
6. What are the characteristics of your family that hinder the care-
9. Which family member would "understand" if you had a brain injury? If you had AIDS?

10. Who would not be able to understand? Why?
11. Who in your family would be least able to cope with or adapt to illness?

REFERENCES

Allen, K., Linn, R., Gutierrez, H., & Willer, M. (1994). Family burden following traumatic brain injury. *Rehabilitation Psychology, 39,* 29–48.

Armstrong, C. (1991). Emotional changes following brain injury: Psychological and neurological components of depression, denial, and anxiety. *Journal of Rehabilitation,* April/May/June, 15–21.

Bader, J. L., & Robbins, R. (2001). *Good grief!: Helping families cope.* Washington, D.C.City, ST: Alexander Graham Bell Association for the Deaf and Hard of Hearing, Inc.

Blacher, J. (1984). Sequential stages of adjustment to the birth of a child with handicaps: Fact or artifact? *Mental Retardation, 22*(2), 55–68.

Blackford, K. A. (1999). A child's growing up with a parent who has multiple sclerosis: Theories and experiences. *Disability and Society, 14*(5), 673–685.

Bramlett, R., Hall, J., Barnett, D., & Rowell, R. (1995). Child development/educational status in kindergarten and family coping as predictors of parenting stress: Issues for parent consultation. *Journal of Psycho-educational Assessment, 13,* 157–166.

Bray, G. P. (1977). Reactive patterns in families of the severely disabled. *Rehabilitation Counseling Bulletin,* March, 236–239.

Caplan, E. (1976). The family as a support system. In E. Caplan & M. Killilen (Eds.), *Support systems and mutual help.* New York: Grune and Stratton.

Carter, R. T., & Cook, R. T. (1991). A culturally relevant perspective for understanding the career paths of visible racial/ethnic group people. In Z. Leibowitz & D. Lea (Eds.), *Adult career development.* Washington, DC: National Career Development Association.

Caroff, P., & Mailick, M. D. (1985). The patient has a family: Reaffirming social work's domain. *Health and Social Work, 10,* 17–34.

Cavallo, M., & Savcedo, C. (1995). Traumatic brain injury in families from culturally diverse populations. *Journal of Head Trauma Rehabilitation, 10,* 66–77.

Chan, R. (2000). Stress and coping in spouses of persons with spinal cord injuries. *Clinical Rehabilitation, 14*(2), 137–144.

Chwallisz, K. (1992). Perceived stress and caregiver burden after brain injury: A theoretical integration. *Rehabilitation Psychology, 37,* 189–201.

Cohen, M. S. (1999). Families coping with childhood chronic illness: A research review. *Family Systems and Health, 17*(2), 149–163.

Curtiss, G., Klemz, S., & Vanderploeg, R. D. (2000). Acute impact of severe traumatic brain injury on family structure and coping responses. *Journal of Head Trauma Rehabilitation, 15*(5), 1113–1122.

Dell Orto, A. E., & Power, P. W. (1994). *Head injury and the family: A life and living perspective.* Winter Park, FL: PMD Publishers Group, Inc.

Dillard, J. M. (1983). *Multi-cultural counseling.* Chicago: Nelson Hall.

Epperson, M. (1977). Families in sudden crisis. *Social Work in Health Care, 2-3*, 265–273.

Faulkner, R. A. & Davey, M. (2002). Children and adolescents of cancer patients: The impact of cancer on the family. *The American Journal of Family Therapy, 30*, 63–72.

Ferguson, P. M. (2002). A place in the family: An historical interpretation of research on parental reactions to having a child with a disability. *Journal of Special Education, 36*(3), 124–130.

Giaquinta, B. (1977). Helping families face the crisis of cancer. *American Journal of Nursing,* October, 1585–1588.

Harry, B. (2002). Trends and issues in serving culturally diverse families of children with disabilities. *The Journal of Special Education, 36*(3), 131–138.

Hampton, N. Z., & Marshall, S. A. (2000). Culture, gender, self-efficacy, and life satisfaction: A comparison between Americans and Chinese people with spinal cord injuries. *Journal of Rehabilitation, 66*(3), 21–28.

Keydel, C. (1988). The impact of a handicapped child on adolescent siblings: Implications for professional intervention. In P. W. Power, A. E. Dell Orto, & M.B. Gibbons, *Family interventions throughout chronic illness and disability.* New York: Springer Publishing.

Keydel, C. F. (1991). *An exploration of perception and coping behaviors in family members living with a closed-head-injured relative.* Unpublished manuscript.

Knox, M., Parmester, T., Atkinson, N., & Yazbeck, M. (2000). Family control: The views of families who have a child with an intellectual disability. *Journal of Applied Research in Intellectual Disabilities, 13*, 17–28.

Kolakowsky-Hayner, S. A., Miner, K. D., & Kreutzer, J. S. (2001). Long-term life quality and family needs after traumatic brain injury. *Journal of Head Trauma Rehabilitation, 16*(4), 374–385.

Kosciulek, J. (1994). Relationship of family coping with head injury to family adaptation. *Rehabilitation Psychology, 39*, 215–230.

Kreutzer, J., Devany, C., & Bergquist, S. (1994). Family needs following brain injury: A quantitative analysis. *Journal of Head Trauma Rehabilitation, 9*, 104–115.

Kübler-Ross, E. (1969). *On death and dying.* New York: MacMillan & Co.

Lin, S. L. (2000). Coping and adaptation in families of children with cerebral palsy. *Exceptional Children, 66*(2), 201–218.

Livneh, H. (2001). Psychosocial adaptation to chronic illness and disability: A conceptual framework. *Rehabilitation Counseling Bulletin, 44*(3), 151–160.

Lustig, D. C. (1999). Family caregiving of adults with mental retardation: Key issues for rehabilitation counselors. *Journal of Rehabilitation, 65*(2), 26–35.

Lustig, D. C. (2002). Family coping in families with a child with a disability. *Education and Training in Mental Retardation and Developmental Disabilities, 37*(1), 14–22.

MacFarlene, M. (1999). Treating brain-injured clients and their families. *Family Therapy, 26*, 13–30.

Mathis, M. (1984). Personal needs of family members of critically ill patients with and without acute brain injury. *Journal of Neurosurgical Nursing, 16*, 36–44.

Mitiguy, J.S. (1990) Coping with survival. *Headlines*, 228.

Muscott, H. S. (2002). Exceptional partnerships: Listening to the voices of families. *Preventing School Failure, 46*(2), 66–67.

Olson, D. H., McCubbin, H. I., Barnes, H., Larsen, A., Muxen, M., & Wilson, M. (1983). *Families: What makes them work?* Beverly Hills, CA: Sage.

Orsillo, S. M., McCaffrey, R. J., & Fisher, J. M. (1993). Siblings of head-injured individuals: A population at risk. *Journal of Head Trauma Rehabilitation, 8*(1), 102–115.

Palmer, S., Kriegsman, K. & Palmer, J. B. (2000). *Spinal cord injury. A guide for living.* Baltimore, MD: Johns Hopkins University Press.

Pearlin, L. I., & Schooler, C. (1978). The structure of coping. *Journal of Health and Human Behavior, 19*, 2-21.

Power, P. W. (1991). Family coping with chronic illness and rehabilitation. In F. K. Judd, G. D. Burrows, & D. R. Lipsitt (Eds). *Handbook on General Hospital Psychiatry*, Amsterdam: Elsever Publishers.

Power, P. E. (1995). Family. In A. E. Dell Orto & R. P. Marinelli (Eds). *The encyclopedia of disability and rehabilitation.* New York: Simon & Schuster/MacMillan.

Rape. R. N., Bush, J. P., & Slavin, L. A. (1992). Toward a conceptualization of the family's adaptation to a member's brain injury: A critique of developmental stage models. *Rehabilitation Psychology, 37*(1), 3–22.

Rogers-Dulon, J., & Blacher, J. (1995). African-American families, religion, and disability: A conceptual framework. *Mental Retardation, 33*(4), 226–238.

Rolland, J. (1994). *Families, illness and disability.* New York: Basic Books.

Santana, S., & Santana, D. (2001). *An introduction to Mexican culture for rehabilitation service providers.* Buffalo, NY: Center for International Rehabilitation Research Information and Exchange.

Scorgie, K., Wilgosh, L., & McDonald, L. (1996). A qualitative study of managing life when a child has a disability. *Developmental Disabilities Bulletin, 24*, 69–90.

Stebbins, P., & Leung, P. (1998). Changing family needs after brain injury. *Journal of Rehabilitation, 64*(4), 15–22.

Urbach, J. R., Sonenklar, N. A., & Culbart, J. P. (1994). Risk factors and assessment in children of brain-injured parents. *Journal of Neuropsychiatry, 6*(3), 289–295.

Waaland, P. K., & Kreutzer, J. S. (1988). Family response to childhood traumatic brain injury. *Journal of Head Trauma Rehabilitation, 3*(4), 51–63.

Weihs, K., Fisher, L., & Baird, M. (2002). Families, health, and behavior. *Family Systems and Health, 20*(1), 7–46.

Williams, J. M., & Kay, T. (1991). *Brain injury: A family matter.* Baltimore, MD: Paul H. Brookes Publishing Company.

Zeigler, E. A. (1987). Spouses of persons who are brain injured: Overlooked victims. *Journal of Rehabilitation, 53*, 50–53.

Part II

Family Interventions

An evolving challenge for health and human care personnel, as well as the systems in which they work, is to become more aware of and responsive to the needs of families transformed by the demands of the illness and disability experience (Baird, 2002; Bush & Pargament, 1997). But Connell and Connell (1995) believe that "obstacles to coping and recovery exist if medical personnel perceive the illness differently from the patient or the family" (p. 30). This lack of common ground often adds to the stress and strain experienced by the family forced many times to renegotiate a relationship with the family member who may be quite different from the person they knew, loved, and/or cared for prior to the onset of the chronic illness or severe disability.

Further, families and human care professionals are frequently caught between managed care and managed cost, often resulting in "mangled care" that may solve problems for some but may create problems for others. Because of these issues, all rehabilitation professionals face a daunting responsibility in assisting family members to weave their way through complex medical and insurance systems. A necessary component for beginning this difficult task is for the family to receive timely, relevant attention to their needs, and an intervention that includes an understanding of their needs and provides appropriate support, imparts insightful coping strategies, alerts them to available resources, and urges family members to take good care of themselves. All of these assistive ingredients are strategies the family can use to become a vital resource during the treatment and rehabilitation of their family member.

From their review of the literature, Weihs, Fisher, and Baird (2002) report that pre-intervention and intervention research suggests that a family-focused approach to the management of chronic disease should address three overriding goals:

- To help families cope with and manage the continuing stresses inherent in chronic disease management as a team, rather than as individuals
- To mobilize the patient's natural support system to enhance family closeness, increase mutually supportive interactions among family members, and build additional extra familial support to improve disease management and the health and well being of patients and all family members.
- To minimize intrafamilial hostility and criticism, and reduce the adverse effects of external stress and disease-related trauma on family life.

Chapter 5 establishes a diagnostic framework for developing a unique intervention approach in chapter 6. Both chapters consider the work demands of many helping professionals, who usually only have the opportunities for family contact as they pursue their primary professional duties. Chapter 6 also elaborates on assisting families to cope and to utilize the family resources to enhance their own adjustment efforts to the demands of care giving. Effective coping styles could buffer the effects of stressful factors that often impede the family member's attempts to become a useful partner in treatment and rehabilitation.

Chapter 7 adds a further dimension to assisting a family impacted by a chronic disease. When family members become involved in group counseling, they can learn new ways to manage the medical situation and, importantly, discover previously unknown resources for building hope. Chapter 8 introduces into the family literature some needed insights into the family-professional relationship. Frequently, delicate situations arise if the family has misperceptions regarding treatment and rehabilitation outcomes, especially if they diverge greatly from those of the health care team. Existing systems cannot meet all of the expectations of families, but families can have options. Identifying options and choices is integral to effective communication styles between family members and health professionals. These issues are all discussed in chapter 8 .

The personal statements of Louise, a mother, and Sabine underline the importance of effective relationships between the family and health care personnel. Intervention approaches will not be effective unless there is this working alliance, and their stories illustrate what can go awry when all parties are not in harmony concerning treatment goals. Through such collaboration that energizes intervention efforts, families can be helped to deal with the losses created by illness and disability and mobilize their natural support system to become a valuable resource for the family member who is dealing with illness and disability-caused limitations.

REFERENCES

Baird, M. (2002). Comments on the commissioned report of health and behavior: The interplay of biological, behavioral, and societal influences. *Families, Systems, & Health, 20*(1), 1–6.

Bush, E., & Pargament, K. (1997). Family coping with chronic pain. *Family, Systems, & Health, 15*(2), 147–160.

Connell, G. M., & Connell, L. C. (1995). In hospital consultation: Systemic intervention during medical crisis. *Family, Systems, & Health, 13*(1), 29.

Weihs, K., Fisher, L, & Baird, M. (2002). Families, health and behavior: A section of the commissioned report by the committee on health and behavior: Research, practice, and policy. *Families, Systems, & Health, 20*(1), 7–46.

5

An Approach to Family Assessment

The family can be a valuable resource in the treatment and rehabilitation of people with chronic illness or severe disability. Illness and disability are actually a family affair, and the person's adjustment or adaptation is a function of both the person and the family environment (DeJong, Batavia, & Williams, 1990; Durgin, 1989; Schwentor & Brown, 1989). Importantly, an appraisal of what it is in family life that influences the family member experiencing illness or disability can become the basis for the development of appropriate family helping strategies. Family assessment is often a key ingredient for developing an effective management plan (Dell Orto & Power, 1994; Power, Dell Orto, & Gibbons, 1988).

The focus of family assessment has undergone an interesting evolution since 1940. To understand family dynamics, earlier family literature emphasized personal satisfaction and perceptions of relationships within families. Later, identifying the dynamics of pre-marital and marital chances for satisfying adjustment dominated assessment literature. Family-systems thinking currently influences the field. With the focus on family-system relationships, evaluation techniques are now used to pinpoint specific problems in relationships, to obtain information about coping strategies, and to identify resources that could make the adjustment to family changes progress more smoothly (Sporakowski, 1995). To acquire this information, a variety of techniques are available, such as observational methods, genograms, historical approaches, and family adaptation measures (Steinglass, 1979; McGolderick & Gerson, 1985; Masters & Johnson, 1970; Forman & Hagan, 1984; Thomlison, 2002).

This chapter describes the purpose and principles of family assessment, identifies selected, traditional approaches to family evaluation, and then discusses an approach to assessment that is applicable to the different roles and functions of health and allied health professionals. Family assessment is a complex process and is different, both in focus and emphasis, from individual client appraisal. Most health professionals have been trained only to diagnose and understand the person who is ill or disabled. Fortunately, however, today many training programs are assisting future helping professionals to become aware of the difference between "individuals and their family" and "the individual in the family" (Rolland, 1994).

PURPOSE OF FAMILY ASSESSMENT

The goals of family appraisal are usually determined by the job responsibilities and opportunities of the members of the health care team. In other words, the "problem-to-be worked" may be different for each professional. An assessment strategy will be influenced by varied professional responsibilities. If a professional's many job functions, for example, are to focus on family crisis situations, with specific attention to immediate problems and complaints, then information will be organized and synthesized around those issues. A nurse in a medical setting, for example, will focus on the interplay of the family members in relation to the care and treatment of the ill child or adult. A rehabilitation counselor may be more concerned with how family members influence the client's motivation toward the achievement of vocational rehabilitation goals. Social workers and family counselors may often direct their attention to how the family can utilize community support systems for its own survival. Physical or occupational therapists may explore how the family can become a necessary partner of the patient for continuing a treatment regimen at home or in the agency setting.

Many health professionals also may have limited opportunities to work with families. It is not a designated priority among their job functions. In many rehabilitation agencies, the rapid flow of clients through the system usually necessitates short-term attention. Evaluation strategies for families may be shaped by the overall length of time offered to the professional for any family involvement. Because families can often be seen only briefly, family assessment is usually conducted within a short-time framework, and the appraisal approach must be carefully designed to make effective use of the limited assessment opportunity. Whatever the involvement, however, three words are crucial to any family assessment: identifying, understanding, and planning (Thomlison, 2002).

IDENTIFYING

While the format and content of the family assessment will vary, focus should be on what the family needs and will need at a particular point in time, what services should be provided, and what the obstacles to family adaptation and eventual adjustment are. Further appraisal areas to be explored will depend on the nature of the family problem and the type of family goals ideally to be achieved. Many family assessments, consequently, can be quite comprehensive because of the importance of extensive information to address the problem, or brief because of time restrictions and, as stated earlier, job responsibilities.

UNDERSTANDING

Helping professionals may be skilled in obtaining information from family members. But this information must be organized and then synthesized in order to connect it to identified problem areas. Also, family members should be aware at some time in the assessment process of how all of the information provided by them is relevant to the difficulties they are experiencing or are about to face. Clarification of knowledge gained during a family assessment process must be considered an important issue if families are to be effective partners in eventual treatment and rehabilitation planning for their family member, and if they are to reach adaptive goals.

PLANNING

All the assessment information learned during the family interview, after it is organized and synthesized, should become the foundation for appropriate, family intervention. This information is an essential component of family management and adjustment plans.

PRINCIPLES OF FAMILY ASSESSMENT IN ILLNESS AND DISABILITY-RELATED SITUATIONS

Since the focus of this book is on assisting families both to become effective partners in their family member's treatment and rehabilitation and to organize their resources to meet the challenges related to the chronic illness or disability, there are selective principles that will guide assessment approaches:

1. The family is an interactive system, and change affects all family members (Cohen & Siefker, 1997). As a system, the family lives in a

context and it constantly has exchanges with the social environment. This family system develops boundaries, which serve to define separateness and autonomy in a family and its subsystems (Minuchin, 1974; Rolland, 1994). Family behaviors are usually related to one another (Olson, 2000). During family assessment, consequently, it is important to look beyond an individual's communication or behavior and observe and understand how that expression is influenced by family relationships and interaction.

2.   Family members are experts on their circumstances and experiences (Dell Orto & Power, 1994). During family appraisal every effort must be taken to provide family members with the opportunity not only to answer direct questions, but also to expand on their responses so that feelings and varied perceptions are expressed. Appraisal questions should act as stimuli to further elaboration and shared viewpoints on their family situation.

3.   Family assessments should be an ongoing process because of the nature of illnesses and disabilities a well as the changes in the resources and specific supports that are available to the family. The course of an illness or changes in a disability condition may result, for example, in shifting family roles and perhaps the emergence of many crisis situations (Sander & Kreutzer, 1999). Illness progression can cause a change in family priorities, and information gained during this time may be quite different from what was obtained when family dynamics were first identified at illness diagnosis or disability onset.

4.   Family assessment can be conducted in many ways (Dell Orto & Power, 2000). Standardized and quantifiable methods are traditionally utilized and these approaches employ questionnaires that ask for an individual's perception of the family's functioning (Urbach, Sonenklar, & Culbert, 1994). Other approaches include observing the family in the home when they are carrying out assigned tasks and conducting a family interview in the home setting. An assessment conducted in the home enables the interviewer to evaluate areas such as individual dynamics, family interaction, living arrangements, environment, and resources. With everyone assembled in the home, communication can be encouraged among family members, and the nature of problems arising from the illness or disability can be discussed openly. In their own environment, family members are usually more open to the interviewer, more prone to discuss their illness/disability-related problems, and more ready to share information. However, there must be consideration given to cultural and familial values and traditions that may limit the amount of discussion of family issues and problems with someone who is not a family member. But if possible, all family members who are

living in the home or who have almost immediate availability to the family home should be included when the interview is conducted. At the beginning of any family assessment, the interviewer may be unaware of those persons who have a decided influence on the management of the person with an illness or disability. Someone who is missing from the assessment interview could be the very person who has a dominating influence on the client or the family process, and who could influence treatment and rehabilitation outcomes.

5.   A family's culture usually impacts their role functioning, decision-making, and the manner they use support resources (Thomlison, 2002). Each family has a distinct way of thinking and communicating, and family assessment should consider cultural, ethnic, and gender orientation (Harry, 2002). These orientations also shape family values, and such values may be guideposts for family adaptive patterns.

6.   With the information to be obtained during family appraisal, a perspective that can be very useful when assisting families to adjust to changes emerging from a medical trauma is the identification of family strengths. When family members are experiencing their personal and collective traumas when responding to a severe illness or disability, these assets may be ignored or forgotten. Most of the assessment approaches to family dynamics have emphasized pathological or dysfunctional characteristics of the family unit (Thomlison, 2002; Wilcoxon, 1985). But the identification of family strengths can pinpoint family resources, serve as reinforcements for family members, and indicate "markers" for intervention. Some of these family strengths are the following:

a)   Ability of the family to listen
b)   Shared perceptions of reality
c)   Ability to take responsibility for illness/disability-related problems
d)   Ability to use negotiation in family problem solving
e)   Willingness to take good care of themselves
f)   Ability to focus on the present, rather than on only past events or disappointments
g)   Ability to discuss their concerns
h)   Ability to provide positive reinforcements to each other
i)   Willingness to have hope and to appreciate that change is possible.

SELECTED FAMILY ASSESSMENT APPROACHES

When a family is experiencing the impact of a sudden injury or unexpected diagnosis, or when they are confronted with adjustment concerns during the long course of treatment or rehabilitation, the process of family assessment to pinpoint selected issues presents unique demands. To respond to these demands Rolland (1994) has identified the appraisal areas of family communication, intimacy, rebalancing relationship skews, e.g., "my" versus "our" problem, caregiver roles, and establishing healthy boundaries as important target issues to explore. In illness and disability-related family situations, these areas provide a helpful structure for the assessment process. However, a better understanding of how these focused areas interact with each other in the family context can be gained by briefly reviewing two traditional approaches to family assessment. Neither approach was developed primarily for evaluating family dynamics in illness or disability situations. But the concepts identified in these two models and those formulated by Rolland (1994) re-energize each other and provide a foundation for which interview questions are developed for family assessment at certain points in time from initial onset through outpatient status of the illness or disability. These questions will be described later in this chapter.

The two models of family appraisal are the Circumplex Model of Marital and Family Systems described by Olson (2000), and the McMaster Approach to Families, outlined by Miller, Ryan, Keitner, Bishop, and Epstein (2000). The Circumplex Model is particularly in harmony with the principles of family assessment identified earlier in this chapter.

CIRCUMPLEX MODEL

This approach, described most recently by Olson (2000), and building on his earlier writings, is system-focused and integrates three dimensions that can be considered relevant to understanding dynamics for those family members who are living with a chronic illness or severe disability. These dimensions are family cohesion, flexibility, and communication. Family cohesion refers to the emotional bonding that family members have toward one another. Such factors as coalitions between family members, time, space, friends, decision-making, interests, and recreation are all concepts that can be used to evaluate this cohesion. Apart from the quality of family relationship patterns prior to disease or disability onset, the impact of a medical event can challenge family connections to each other. As discussed in an earlier chapter, family members may have their own unique response to the situation, and the emotional responses may fuel behaviors of disengagement or connection, or even enmeshment. Within an enmeshed relationship there is an intense amount of emotional closeness (Olson, 2000). Such a relationship can foster high levels of dependence among family members. Personal energy is then directed within the family rather than necessarily exploring available resources outside of the family. It is important to note, however, that in some family situations enmeshment can be more of an asset than a liability. When there are few available external resources, for example, emotional closeness among family members may serve as a coping strategy. Because of its implications for family adaptation to an illness or disability experience, cohesion could be explored during assessment as a significant resource for the possibility of reaching appropriate adjustment goals.

Family flexibility, another dimension in this model, is defined as the amount of change in family leadership and role relationships that occurs when some disruption occurs. A family appraisal approach should include how the family is reacting to the many illness or disability-related changes or situational stressors. The focus of understanding flexibility is how the family can balance its everyday functioning with necessary changes. If, during the course of an illness or disability, the family can maintain some balance through negotiation and open decision-making, then the family as a unit can be more functional over time (Olson, 2000). When family roles are shared and there is fluid change at each trigger point of treatment and rehabilitation, then individuals have the potential to become resilient during these perceived disruptions in family life.

Family communication includes family members' ability to listen to each other, to self-disclose, to speak clearly about personal needs and expectations, and to respect each other. When a family is traumatized by an illness or disability, members often "shut down," refusing to speak about the event or even communicate personal fears, needs, and expectations. The family, of course, should not be expected to respond in ideal ways, but an open discussion of feelings, hopes, and concerns can provide an atmosphere where family problem solving can happen without acrimony and with the resolve to do what is best at a particular time. To learn how family members speak to each other can provide useful insights into how a family can maximize its resources and partner with the ill or disabled member for treatment and rehabilitation goals.

It is expected that family systems will change in response to illness and disability. The three dimensions of the Circumplex Model can suggest whether families have the resources to shift their system and what is the most appropriate way to manage the losses, changes, and adjustments in family life effectively.

McMaster Approach

This model is also based on systems theory, but covers a number of dimensions that are useful when identifying family dynamics challenged by illness and disability transitions experienced by a family member. There are six operational dimensions of family life in the context of family changes: problem solving, communication, roles, affective responsiveness, affective involvement, and behavior control (Miller, Ryan, Keitner, Bishop, & Epstein , 2000). Problem-solving refers to the family's ability to manage problems at a level that sustains effective family functioning; communication conveys an understanding of how information is exchanged within a family; roles are the recurrent patterns of behavior by which individuals meet necessary and other family tasks; affective responsiveness asks the questions: "Do family members respond with a wide range of feelings to a specific, situational context?" and "Is such a response in harmony with the nature of the situation?"; affective involvement refers to the degree to which the family as a whole shows interest in and values the life of individual family members; and behavior control is defined as the pattern of behavior the family displays in crisis, in customary family life, and in interpersonal situations (Miller, Ryan, Keitner, Bishop, & Epstein , 2000).

Family measurement scales have been developed from these six dimensions, e.g., the Family Assessment Device and the McMaster Clinical Rating Scale, and their use requires specialized training. These scales are used occasionally to predict future family adjustment to a variety of chronic illnesses (Bishop, et al., 1987; Kreutzer, Devany, & Bergquist, 1994). For the health professional who is confronted with the immediate responsibility to conduct a family assessment, and for varied reasons cannot use these scales, the six dimensions can provide focus areas for family appraisal, especially in disability and illness situations. The dimension of problem solving, for example, is essential to explore when the family is undergoing a long process of adaptation to the medical event. Though solutions may be elusive, the capacity and existence of family problem-solving skills establishes a foundation for appropriate coping and perhaps eventual resolution.

Both models, consequently, provide many of the constructs for creating an assessment approach that can be used in a variety of settings. The setting for the assessment interview itself can have a decided influence on whether family members feel comfortable or not in providing information. For the nurse or physical therapist, for example, while maintaining confidentiality as much as possible, knowledge of the family may be obtained in a hospital clinic waiting room or in a rehabilitation setting. Social workers, psychiatric nurses, or rehabilitation counselors may utilize an office to make a family appraisal, but the authors believe that, when possible, an effective assessment can be achieved during a family home visit. Family mealtimes, for example have a broad appeal as a source of information. Minuchin, Roseman, and Baker (1978) have done some original work on family luncheons with anorexics and their families. He has attempted to deal with underlying family dysfunctions and utilizes mealtimes to capture some of these family dynamics. Grossman, Pozanski, and Banegas (1983) have also used the family luncheon, whether in the home, in a hospital cafeteria, or a picnic area, to study family interactions. They believe that observation of the family luncheon is a supplement to clinical observations, and is a valuable tool to learn about family dynamics. In these informal settings, families appear to relax more easily and thus a more valid portrait of the family is often obtained. Yet, if the helping professional is sensitive to preserving confidentiality and is attuned to the importance of learning about the family in order to plan effective treatment, then almost any opportunity or place where the family is present can be advantageous for appraisal.

AN APPROACH TO FAMILY ASSESSMENT

The approach now to be explained suggests the development of needed family information, dynamics, skills, and existing family strengths at three trigger points, i.e., the family member's initial treatment, in-hospital medical care, and out-patient status for continued treatment and rehabilitation. Occasionally assessment information may need to be obtained at one trigger point because of family and illness-related circumstances, or if there are only one or possibly two opportunities for a family meeting. Whatever the number of assessment occasions, the interviews are goal-oriented conversations between the interviewer and the family. There are also a number of factors that shape the content and process of the appraisal session. Time constraints, the professional's style of communication, and the family's comfort level are just three of the many influences on the process of the family evaluation. Each interview will be unique, but at the family meeting that is primarily focused on gathering information, there are usually three steps:

STEP 1. MEETING THE FAMILY

The first interaction with family members, regardless of the setting, involves a greeting, perhaps a brief period of social conversation, and an explanation of the purpose of the meeting. It is important to note that all family members may not be present but may become involved at a later time. Throughout the introductions the health professional needs to exercise such basic communication skills as (a) attentiveness, (b) a nonjudgmental attitude, (c) using understandable words when talking with family members, and (d) using verbal re-enforcers such as "I see" or "Yes". Because family members are experiencing the impact of an individual's disability/illness on various emotional levels, this initial meeting may be quite threatening and they may not wish to openly express their feelings. Cultural beliefs influence family communication styles (Hampton & Marshall, 2000; Stanhope, 2002). Yet establishing a tone that conveys respect for these feelings and attitudes, assuring privacy and confidentiality, and being honest, empathic, willing to listen, and direct could be encouraging to the family and help them to achieve a comfort level that could facilitate a productive interaction. Moments or periods of silence and reflection need to be permitted, since they may help family members to organize their thoughts. Importantly, during this introductory period, family interaction styles and language should be observed, while the interviewer also keeps in mind such questions as "Who appear to be the key decisions makers in the family?" and "What is the family's expectation of help seeking and intervention?" Finding an answer to these questions early in the process of family assessment provides both an understanding of family structure and possible resources for assistance in family intervention.

STEP 2. EXPLORING FAMILY REACTIONS, PROBLEMS, STRENGTHS, NEEDS, EXPECTATIONS, AND OTHER DYNAMICS RELATED TO THE ILLNESS/DISABILITY DURING SPECIFIC "TRIGGER" POINTS

This step in the family interview involves asking specific questions related to the particular "trigger point' during the course of the illness or disability. The health and human care professional should not assume anything, and should ask only what he or she believes the family member can answer so that the person feels competent and productive. This communication may be difficult and one should proceed cautiously, exploring carefully family perceptions of what has happened or what they need at the particular time. Also, the helper should ask questions that family members can handle emotionally at the time. In other words, an atmosphere must be created during the family meeting in which people can, perhaps for the first time, risk sharing their emotions and seek information about their concerns.

Of relevance to this step of the family assessment interview is the increasing use of "interventive" questions to identify the impact of a sudden trauma and the possible, resulting changes in family functioning (Wright & Leahey, 1994). Interventive questions are usually of two types: linear and circular (Tomm, 1984). Linear questions explore an individual's descriptions and perceptions of a family concern, are used to gather information, and the focus is on cause and effect. They can begin with such words as "When did ... " or "How much does ... " These questions tend to be constraining, while circular questions are generative, and tend to suggest directions for behavioral change. They also seek connections between individuals, events, or beliefs. They can begin with such phrases as "Who in the family is more ... ", "What's the best advice you have obtained about ... ", "What do you think will happen if ... ", "What do you feel when ... ", and "How much longer will it be before ... ". Both linear and circular questions are used in the proposed approach when the interviewer attempts to gather information at specific periods or "trigger points," of the family member's treatment and rehabilitation.

Trigger Point A: Diagnosis/Beginning of Treatment

Assessment at this particular time is usually brief and can have a crisis intervention orientation. For family members it can be a period of intense anxiety, uncertainty about the future, and accompanying feelings of helplessness, guilt, anger, as well as hope, whether it is realistic or not. The following questions explore family life areas and may provide information leading to potential support:

- What kind of services would be most helpful to you right now?
- Do you have relatives living nearby and available during this time?
- How can I be most helpful to you at this time?
- Have there been any previous crises in the family, and how were they handled?
- What information do you have about what has happened?
- When you found out about the disability or illness, what did you do as a family?
- What is your understanding of what has happened?

Trigger Point B: During the Course of In-hospital Treatment/Rehabilitation

As beginning treatment plans are unfolding at this crucial time in the family member's illness or disability, there are many areas for the health and human care team members to explore. Usually there is more time to discuss family dynamics in relation to the medical situation, and long-term intervention plans can be initially formulated. Each question is directed to the development of these intervention approaches. For many families this meeting may be the first opportunity to discuss family dynamics and changes that are occurring because of the illness/disability event. The following are some questions related to this process:

- Can you describe your family life since the occurrence of the disability illness?
- What information do you now have about the medical condition? What would you like to know?
- What are the differences in your family life since illness/disability onset? What important changes have occurred?
- What is your perceived threat to family functioning because of the disability?
- What are your family needs during the in-hospital stay of your family members?
- Are there other serious family problems or expected problems (e.g., alcoholism, drug abuse, mental illness, or other stressors)? Are they connected with your family member's medical situation?
- Is there communication with extended family or significant others?
- What do you believe is the emotional reaction of your family member who is now undergoing treatment?
- What are the resources available to you?
- What questions do you have of the health professionals who are directly involved with caring for your family member? Do you feel comfortable when communicating with these people?

Trigger Point C: Outpatient Status and Continued Treatment and Rehabilitation

After the family member leaves the hospital, the family has the opportunity to take a vital part in this person's treatment/rehabilitation and eventual adjustment. The family assessment interview is directed towards this family role. The meeting also provides a focus for what the family needs to do to achieve their own adaptation. It is to be noted that this family meeting does not usually explore in-depth such family dynamics as complex communication patterns and lingering unfinished business among family members. Such an exploration may be beyond the time or training provided to the health professional.

The professional realizes, however, that engaging family members in a discussion of their needs and concerns can make a difference in the family member's adjustment and perhaps the family's own quality of life. Following the family greeting, when a beginning alliance of mutual trust and respect is established, an exploration at this trigger point of particular illness/disability-related family dynamics can elicit information on what the family can do to help their family member and themselves:

- Who will be the family member mainly responsible for the "care" of the person is ill or disabled?
- Have new disruptions occurred within the family since hospital discharge?
- Has your relationship to health care providers changed?
- What expectations do you have for your family member who is ill or disabled, and for each other?
- How do you feel about having your family member at home? Do you foresee any problems?
- Have your family needs changed now that he/she is an outpatient?
- What services do you need?
- What is family life going to be like, now that your family member has been discharged from the hospital?
- What do you feel is the most difficult problem for your family at the present time?
- What activities do family members share together?
- Do individual schedules permit much time together at home as a family?
- How would you describe the sibling relationships in your family?
- What do you perceive as your family strengths?
- What information do you have on the capabilities and limitations of your family member who is ill or disabled, especially emotionally, physically, intellectually, and vocationally?
- What do you think are the attitudes of extended family members and close friends about your family member?
- What have you found helpful so far in adapting to your family member who is ill or disabled?
- Is there a great deal of shame, guilt, or feelings of frustration among family members?
- What areas of your family life appear less stressed, strained, or damaged? What areas are most stressed, strained, or damaged?
- What are your beliefs about continuing your role responsibilities in the home and in the world of work?

- Are community agencies available and used? Do they seem to be adequate?

3: Understanding Strengths and Problem Areas for Family and Family Member Adjustment

The health professional should synthesize the collected information and communicate highlights of the family meetings. This information can lead to developing a plan of action to achieve mutual family goals. The relevant family members need to understand these highlights and observations provided by the health care professional. The interviewer not only identifies those family areas that need to be addressed for effective partnering in the family member's treatment and rehabilitation, but also helps the family to rediscover their strengths and the support systems needed for their own stabilization and adjustment. Frequently, suggestions and advice are helpful if the family requests and wants them, is ready to listen, and has the capability to follow these suggestions

Health professionals will often encounter problems that may exceed their abilities or time constraints and that require a referral to another professional, such as a family therapist, a social worker, psychiatrist, or a psychologist particularly trained in the remediation of serious family problems. Making a referral has many components, such as having names of these professionals, being familiar with their style and type of therapy, and the special skills of when to suggest a referral and how to followup. The referral process is an important responsibility for the health professional and its success usually requires that he/she has established a trusting relationship with family members.

Thematic to the assessment areas or questions identified in the three proposed "trigger points" are the issues of family communication and expectations, information about the illness or disability, the way the family utilizes external resources, family needs related to the experience, and the changes that have occurred in the family since the onset of the injury. Information emerging from these issues also assists in the identification of problem areas relevant both to the adjustment of the family and overall life adaptation of the person experiencing physical or emotional changes.

Specific to understanding dynamics relevant to the impact of illness or disability is the realization that information requested from family members may be influenced by ethnic and cultural factors. For example, some information may not be shared because family members believe it to be a private family matter, or "bad luck" to do so. For many ethnic groups disability is a cultural concept, and those needs and concerns that may be significant for one ethnic group may not be for another (Stanhope, 2002). Some ethnic groups may use the extended family as an expected resource in times of crisis or transition while for other cultural groups extended family may simply be unavailable or may not even be asked to provide support. Within each ethnic group there are also intragroup differences and a diversity determined by cultural history and values, social-political conditions, social environments, and economic conditions. Importantly, acculturation issues that can influence family values and response patterns to illness and disability need to be identified for they may suggest the family's willingness to participate in treatment planning (Barnhart, 2001).

CONCLUSION

The three steps in the proposed model of family assessment provide a structure for learning necessary information that then becomes the basis for an intervention approach. Yet, besides the suggested questions that could be asked during the family meetings at each of the time periods identified in this chapter, there are two other assessment tools which can elicit important appraisal information. A family genogram, for example, can be used to collect and organize data that shows intergenerational relationships, conflicts, and supports, to highlight the family history of chronic illnesses or disabilities, and then to portray how family members have managed these medical situations (McGoldrick & Gerson, 1985). Information displaying the family's historical patterns is drawn using symbols. With these symbols various details of family history are depicted indicating significant events. Each event can also become useful to show health professionals and family members intergenerational coping themes (Rolland, 1994). Recreating in a genogram a family history that focuses on illness and disability may further identify connections and significant, recurrent issues related to family strengths and adjustment concerns. Thomlison (2002), citing Wright and Leahey (1994), writes that "The family genogram provides four times as much social, health, family history, and family structural and relational patterns as interviews" (p. 62).

The ecomap (Thomlison, 2002), another approach to gathering information during the family meeting, represents the family's interaction with such systems as extended family, school, work, church, and friends. A circle depicts each of these systems, and lines drawn between these figures and the family indicate the degree of social support available from each resource, as perceived by individual family members. Eco-maps can help to identify the resources to be utilized for managing family stressors during the family's process of adjustment to an illness or disability.

There are several ways, consequently, to conduct a family assessment. Many measures that explore family functioning and that are relevant to illness/disability situations have been developed. The Family Coping Inventory, developed by McCubbin, Boss, Wilson, and Dahl (1991) is a 70-item measure of responses to family stress. The Family Hardiness Index (McCubin, McCubbin, & Thompson, 1991) explores the amount of control of life events that family members perceive they have. Of course, the health care professional should be familiar with the measure, explain the importance and purpose of the measure, be certain that the measure is culturally sensitive and gender bias free, and provide feedback information to family members (Thomlison, 2002). All in all, however, the evaluation will vary both as to extensiveness and subject matter. Family needs will also change as adjustment attempts are made during the different phases of the family member's treatment and rehabilitation.

There are many challenges, moreover, when developing a viable and engaging assessment plan for families who are living with the impact of a severe medical condition. Family members, for example, may have difficulty answering clearly and specifically the requested information. The interviewer needs to be sensitive to the feelings of family members, and ask them to elaborate on their responses. Also, as stated earlier in this chapter, the family may be resistant to providing any information. Support and reassurance should then be given to help comfort the family during the difficult time of managing their life during the family member's illness. There may be other stressors, moreover, which are not directly related to the medical situation, such as pending unemployment or unexpected financial losses. These issues may become distracting to the family when they are trying to communicate during the appraisal meeting.

Despite these many challenges for the family and health professional, a family assessment helps develop an initial connection to the family. The approach described in this chapter is responsive to the many influences that confront, at critical times during treatment and rehabilitation, both the total family system and the family member who has the illness or disability. The next chapter will discuss an intervention approach emerging from the family assessment.

ONE MORE BURDEN: A MOTHER'S PERSPECTIVE

There are many approaches to identifying how a family has been affected by a disability or chronic illness. Frequently the most appropriate and effective way to learn about family dynamics and the family experience of managing an intense medical event is to have a family member write or talk about his/her living situation. From this account many issues can be identified that could form the basis for timely information. The following personal statement presents the challenges faced by a mother whose dreams were shattered. It also highlights her emotional responses to her daughter's disability and illustrates the changing nature of these reactions.

I am a 51-year-old black woman who lives with my daughter in a small house in a quiet section of a southern city. My husband passed away many years ago. I worked as a kitchen helper for many years, but have been unemployed because of serious illnesses and disabilities. I suffer from asthma and a heart condition and receive social security disability insurance (SSDI). I walk with great difficulty and I am not able to go up the stairs in my home. I have two other daughters who live nearby. One has completed the 11th grade and the other has completed 9th. Both are unemployed and receiving aid to families with dependent children (AFDC) because they have children of their own. Both daughters and their children were living with me until the serious accident of my third daughter.

My daughter, 25, was driving when she was hit from behind by a car that ran a stop light, and she was thrown into the windshield. She was not wearing her seatbelt at the time of the accident, and she suffered a serious brain injury. She spent many months in the hospital. When they discharged her, she came to live with me, and my two daughters had to move out. Since she has been at home, she has been unemployed and has received medical certification that she is permanently disabled and unemployable. She tells me that she has a short-term memory impairment and she has frequent seizures, which really scares me. All of my family members are Baptists and we have strong religious beliefs, so I know God will get us through this. My daughter has tried to work for short periods of time, but has been unable to do so because of severe memory problems.

Before the accident, my daughter was a very good girl; she had a great job and her own apartment and she was dating. (The man eventually left her after the accident.) She was also involved in gospel singing at her church. Now all my daughter can do is help me around the house. My other daughters come over quite frequently to see us, and I think they are resentful of her because they had to move out when she left the hospital. Because of my sickness, I was unable to manage all of them under the same roof.

None of the family members believe that my daughter was at fault for the accident, though they all wonder why she was not wearing her seatbelt at the time. I remember telling her the morning of the accident that she should always wear her seatbelt, even if she were driving close to home. If she had done all of this, this accident might not have happened and she would not be limited as she is now, but I guess we all truly believe that the accident just happened and not for any reason. Regardless, all of us know that she was such a good person before the accident. We were very impressed with her lifestyle—a nice apartment with fine furniture and plants everywhere. In our eyes, she was a successful, yet quiet person. Now after the accident she is thinner and even more energetic. Yet I don't say "energetic" in a positive sense. She really has changed for the worse. I still think my daughter is attractive, hopeful, caring, and friendly, but my other daughters think she is more irritable and even a troublemaker. They think that, though she is not the youngest, now she acts like she is the baby in the family. My injured daughter does not share in these beliefs; she feels that she has not changed that much, though she does realize that she is more dependent on all of us, and she has even said that she is less attractive now. After living with my daughter now for several months, I don't think she is going to change too much. We all hope that she will get much better, but I wonder about that.

The most stressful part of our family life now is living with the seizures. We just can't do anything about them, and I worry that they might be fatal and that I might have a heart attack because of the stress. When I get upset, I get chest pains. When we are all here and she has a seizure, we pray together that she will come out of it. Though we panic, we know enough to roll her over from side to side to keep her from swallowing her tongue. Because these seizures happen, and I have a hard time managing them, my daughters come over often just in case. I do get a "funny feeling" when a seizure happens, and I had that feeling the day of the accident. I expect the seizures will get worse, and I don't know what I can do about it. But my many friends and my church have been a support to me during this trial.

Deep down I think it is good for me to have my daughter at home. My friends also seem to visit often. I am happy if my children are all right, and right now I am not so happy because of this brain injury business. I believe that families should take care of each other. I took care of my mother when she was dying and I expect my children will take care of me just as I cared for them. I can manage if we have this togetherness. The doctors are necessary, but it is family that really counts. Though these seizures are getting the best of us, we just group together and do the best we can. God will take care of us.

DISCUSSION QUESTIONS

1. Reflecting on the assessment approach discussed in this chapter, what important issues emerge in this personal statement? How can these issues be used when developing a long-range plan that meets the needs of the mother and daughter?

2. What are the unique stresses related to caring for the daughter at home?

3. Identify the coping resources apparently available to the mother while she is attempting to manage her care giving responsibilities.
4. Would a genogram as an approach to family assessment be useful for planning intervention strategies for this family?
5. How can traditions and cultural expectations be an asset or a liability?

SET 5: PRIME OF LIFE

PERSPECTIVE

Illness and disability rarely occur at a "convenient" time in a person's life. Try to imagine what your life would have been like if you experienced an injury when you were a young adult.

EXPLORATION

1. If you were severely injured would your girlfriend or boyfriend remain with you? What about your husband, wife, mother, father, or significant other?
2. Would you have preferred to be at home or away from home during your rehabilitation?
3. Would your family have responded in a similar or dissimilar manner?
4. What would you have needed to maintain a sense of control, independence, and dignity?
5. Should people who do not wear helmets when riding a motor-cycle be covered by insurance or eligible to sue if injured?
6. How would you respond if your son were brain injured as a result of a motorcycle accident, made great gains, and wanted to buy another motorcycle so he could feel normal again?
7. What is the moral and financial responsibility and liability of a person who gives a ride to someone and they are disabled
8. Do parents have the right to request that a severely brain injured child not be resuscitated? Brought to a hospital? If such a request is made and the child is given medical care over the objections of the parents, who should be responsible for the life-longcare of the child?

REFERENCES

Barnhart, R. C. (2001). Aging adult children with developmental disabilities and their families: Challenges for occupational therapists and physical therapists. *Physical and Occupational Therapy in Pediatrics, 21*(4), 69–81.

Bishop, D., Evans, R., Minden, S., McGowan, M., Marlowe, S., Andreoli, N., Trotter, J., & Williams, C. (1987). Family functioning across different chronic illness/disability groups. *Archives of Physical Medicine and Rehabilitation, 68,* 79–87.

Cohen, M., & Siefker, J. (1997). A family systems approach to rehabilitation counseling. *NARPPS Journal, 12*(3), 94–98.

Dell Orto, A. E., & Power, P. W. (1994). *Head injury and the family: A life and living perspective.* Winter Park, FL: PMD Publishers Group, Inc.

Dell Orto, A. E., & Power, P.W. (2000). *Brain injury and the family,* 2nd ed. Boca Raton, FL: CRC Press.

DeJong, G., Batavia, A. I., & Williams, J. M. (1990). Who is responsible for the lifelong well-being of a person with a brain injury? *Journal of Head Trauma Rehabilitation, 5*(1), 9–22

Durgin, C. J. (1989). Techniques for families to increase their involvement in the rehabilitation process. *Cognitive Rehabilitation,* May-June, 22–25.

Forman, N., & Hagan, B. J. (1984). Measures for evaluating total family functioning. *Family Therapy, XI,* 30–36.

Grossman, J. A., Pozanski, E. O., & Banegas, M. E. (1983). Lunch: Time to study family interactions. *Journal of Psychosocial Nursing and Mental Health Services, 21,* 19–23.

Hampton, N. Z., & Marshall, A. (2000). Culture, gender, self-efficacy, and life satisfaction: A comparison between Americans and Chinese people with spinal cord injuries. *Journal of Rehabilitation, 66*(3), 21–28.

Harry, B. (2002). Trends and issues in serving culturally diverse families of children with disabilities. *The Journal of Special Education, 36*(3), 131–138.

Kreutzer, J., Devany, C., & Bergquist, S. (1994). Family needs following brain injury: A quantitative analysis. *Journal of Head Trauma Rehabilitation, 9,* 104–115.

Masters, W. H., & Johnson, V. E. (1970. *Human sexual inadequacy.* Boston: Little, Brown.

McCubbin, H. I., Boss, P. G., Wilson, L. R., & Dahl, B. B. (1991). Family coping inventory. In H. I. McCubbin & A. I. Thompson (Eds.). *Family assessment inventories for research and practice.* Madison, WI: University of Wisconsin Press.

McCubbin, M. A., McCubbin, H. I., & Thompson, A. I. (1991). Family hardiness index. In H. I. McCubbin & A. I. Thompson (Eds.). *Family assessment inventories for research and practice.* Madison, WI: University of Wisconsin Press.

McGolderick, M., & Gerson, T. (1985). *Genograms in family assessment.* New York: Norton.

Miller, I. W, Ryan, C. E., Keitner, G. I., Bishop, D. S., & Epstein, N. B. (2000). The McMaster approach to families: Theory, assessment, treatment and research. *Journal of Family Therapy, 22,* 168–189.

Minuchin, S. (1974). *Families and family therapy.* Cambridge, MA: Harvard University Press.

Minuchin, S., Roseman, B., & Baker, L. (1978). *Psychosomatic families: Anorexia nervosa in context.* Cambridge, MA: Harvard University Press.

Olson D. H. (2000). Circumplex model of marital and family systems. *Journal of Family Therapy*, 144–167.

Power, P. W., Dell Orto, A. E., & Gibbons, M. B. (1988). *Family interventions throughout chronic illness and disability*. New York: Springer Publishing.

Rolland, J. S. (1994). *Families, illness, and disability*. New York: Basic Books.

Sander, A., & Kreutzer, J. (1999). A holistic approach to family assessment after brain injury. In M. Rosenthal, E. Griffin, J. Kreutzer, & B. Pentland (Eds.) *Rehabilitation of the adult and child with traumatic brain injury*. Philadelphia: F.A. Davis.

Schwentor, D., & Brown, P. (1989). Assessment of families with a traumatically brain-injured relative. *Cognitive Rehabilitation*, 8–14.

Sporakowski, M. (1995). Assessment and diagnosis in marriage and family counseling. *Journal of Counseling and Development, 74*, 60–64.

Stanhope, V. (2002). Culture, control, and family involvement: A comparison of psychosocial rehabilitation in India and the United States. *Psychiatric Rehabilitation Journal, 25*(3), 273–280.

Steinglass, P. (1979). The home observation assessment method (HOAM): Real time naturalistic observation of families in their homes. *Family Process, 18*, 337–354.

Thomlison, B. (2002). *Family assessment handbook*. Pacific Grove, CA: Brooks/Cole.

Tomm, K. (1984). One perspective on the Milan systemic approach: 2. Description of session format, interviewing style, and interventions. *Journal of Marital and Family Therapy, 10*(3), 252–271.

Urbach, J., Sonenklar, N., & Culbert, J. (1994). Risk-factors and assessment in children of brain-injured parents. *Journal of Neuropsychiatry, 6*, 289–295.

Wilcoxon, S.A. (1985). Healthy family functioning: The other side of family pathology. *Journal of Counseling and Development, 63*, 495–498.

Wright, L.M., & Leahey, M. (1994). Calgary family intervention model: One way to think about change. *Journal of Marital and Family Therapy, 20*(4), 381–395.

An Intervention Approach

T he basic premises of this book are that persons with disabilities or illness usually live within a social system called a family and that the condition of one family member influences the quality of life of other family members (Cohen, 1999). With the impact of a medical event the family undergoes a change of roles and frequently a readjustment in their expectations and modification of their hopes, dreams, and aspirations. While playing a vital role in their family member's management of disability/illness-related concerns, at the same time they are often confronted with the challenges of meeting the demands of their own daily responsibilities. But regardless of their demands, priorities, or challenges, the family remains a highly influential component of how the individual member is going to adapt to both treatment and rehabilitation goals (Weihs, Fisher, & Baird, 2002; Power, Dell Orto, & Gibbons, 1988).

Supporting the credibility of these premises is a disability philosophy that fuels the engine of a proposed intervention approach. A traditional view of disability maintains that the occurrence of a disability or illness within a family is primarily and perhaps exclusively a tragedy. The event brings continuing emotional pain and the exclusion from a range of activities by the family, thus creating a disabling environment (Oliver & Sapey, 1999; Priestley, 1999). The belief that is advocated in this book is that the onset of a disability or illness brings choices, the opportunity for a new, enriching family identity, and the chance to take control of how assistance will be provided to all family members during the course of the treatment and rehabilitation process. Swain and French (2000) refer to this belief as the "Affirmation Model of Disability." This approach emphasizes that those with disabilities and their family members have the opportunities to enjoy life, to affirm positive life values, and to determine their own lifestyles. This affirmation belief focuses on what families can do to become resilient while experiencing disability and illness demands, how individual and family strengths can be enhanced, and in what ways family members can be empowered to remain emotionally and physically healthy when confronted with stressful life events. The "Affirmation Model" is a valuing approach. Consequently, intervention strategies to assist the family are then developed by such building mechanisms as empowerment, resilience, and self-determining tools. Affirmation of present experiences and planned expectations becomes a perspective for helping efforts by health professionals and generates intervention goals that make these expectations and experiences accessible (Swain & French, 2000).

This chapter will propose an intervention approach that is generated by these affirmation-influenced goals. To establish the foundation for this specific approach also implies that selective assumptions for intervention be identified. These assumptions will be discussed, followed by a formulation of the goals, and an explanation of the intervention itself. To be noted is that the basis of intervention is in a family context. In the past, the family as a functioning unit has been the target of such helping efforts as psychoeducational strategies, interventions that affect family relationship quality so as to prevent the medical situation from dominating family life, and family therapy. Family therapy includes the attention to such problems as sexual and communication dysfunctions, and control issues (Weihs, Fisher, & Baird, 2002). But the intervention approach outlined in this chapter focuses on particular factors unique and distinct from traditional modalities. The circumstances of time, professional roles, the nature of losses and changes associated with illness and disability, and a different guiding philosophy for helping family members in medical situations all necessitate an approach that responds to the distinctive needs of family members.

ASSUMPTIONS

For an intervention approach to be relevant to the needs and demands of families, certain assumptions are critical for those living with illness or disability:

1. An intervention effort directed toward the person and family is a joint venture shared by health care professionals and family members. If the person, family members, and professional workers share their energy and resources, it will facilitate the attainment of common goals. When they become partners in treatment and rehabilitation efforts, family members generally develop more willingness to work as a team. This is particularly true when family members choose between competing goals and values as they attempt to cope with many severe disabilities

and terminal illnesses. The degree of consensus that develops among family members and health professionals regarding, for example, the ranking of family priorities can become a crucial factor in the family's ability to deal successfully with adjustment demands. What often fosters this consensus is the mutuality that has already been established between the health care worker and the family (Pieper & Singer, 1991).

2.   There will be focused times during the course of treatment and rehabilitation for the family member when families will need specific attention to their needs and other concerns. Each of these "trigger points" must be examined individually because each can bring unique problems. For example, when the person with a disability or illness is at home and undergoing outpatient rehabilitation, caring responsibilities may force family members to assume different roles in the home (Mac-Farlene, 1991).

3.   Families go through levels of changes and shifts in their disability/illness-related needs. The needs for information, maintaining family boundaries, creating personal meaning of what has happened that, in turn, facilitates coping efforts, seeking support, and achieving flexibility in family roles will vary among family members. Additionally, while maintaining communication and cooperation with helping professionals and avoiding burnout, the family's hopes and dreams will emerge in different time periods during treatment and rehabilitation.

4.   The family member's disability or illness is only one of the factors shaping the adaptive or nonadaptive responses of the family. Cultural norms, beliefs, and behaviors influence the family's expectations and perceptions concerning disability/illness-related management issues. Interventions should fit into the family's cultural context. There may be language and value differences between helping professionals and family members. There are also acculturation and racial identity factors that impact on the family's adjustment. These factors may be the lens through which family members perceive the disability and its implications for family life.

5.   There are many family risk factors that should be identified when developing intervention strategies. The lack of available support systems, not understanding the disability or illness and its impact on family functioning, the presence of continued, external stress, role conflicts within the family, and family members' dysfunctional coping approaches, such as denial, role rigidity, and overprotectiveness can each present an obstacle for the helping professional when assisting the family to deal with the medical situation. Also, a pervading presence of anger within the family that is displayed by persistent blame and criticism of other family members can prevent family cohesion, a togeth-

erness that facilitates management efforts, unless there is a viable sup-port system in place. Moreover, single-parent households who may have little access to necessary support systems are vulnerable to serious diffi-culties when attempting to handle care-giving responsibilities.

6.   Many families will be quite resistant to any intervention attempts by health and human care professionals. The availability of secondary gain factors, e.g., financial advantages, increased attention to the family, and opportunities for family member reconciliation because of an illness or disability, may convince the family that any outside assistance that would change their present situation would not be welcome or add any particular benefit and, in effect, could make the situation worse. For many reasons the family members are comfortable with the new "status quo," and they perceive any intervention as a threat to the perceived gains from the illness or disability.

7.   When there is family participation in developing helping plans, intervention efforts can facilitate a renewed family identity that empha-sizes individual responsibility, an awareness of more comprehensive choices, and self-determination. What may influence family involvement are the changing dynamics of an individual family, changing priorities, and the type and severity of the family member's disability. Many families need some form of partnership that will provide the family with a shared responsibility for their family member's adjustment and rehabilitation. This partnership can include education and perhaps training. This involvement will more easily be achieved if family input is welcomed and encouraged from the beginning of treatment. Becoming involved prompts the family to discuss new ideas and strategies before decision-making and intervention takes place.

8.   While intervention may depend on the socioeconomic and edu-cational status of both the family and the person with the illness or disability, it is unrealistic to expect all families to participate at the same level, and passive participation should not be labeled as uncaring. It could be the reflection of family traditions or culture. Also, family intervention is not prescriptive but offers options to assist their family member during the process of adaptation.

INTERVENTION GOALS

Emerging from these assumptions are both overall intervention goals and then specific objectives that may be achieved at designated times when helping family members during the entire disability/illness experi-ence. These times have been identified in earlier chapters as "trigger points." But adaptation to an illness or disability is usually ongoing and adjustment attempts will stimulate varied family reactions and demands. During the unfolding process of care giving efforts, however, there are two overall intervention goals that are in harmony with one of the book's premises, namely, that the family is an important, valuable partner in the person's treatment and rehabilitation.

Intervention Goal #1: Assist Family Members to Adapt to the Illness/ Disability at Specific "Trigger Points."

Intervention Goal #2: Assist the Family to Assist the Family Member with the Illness or Disability Throughout the Treatment and Rehabilitation Process.

These two intervention goals are thematic to the "trigger points." These three times have been identified as critical, because certain needs emerge or important concerns are re-experienced. If these differential needs and concerns are responded to, it can make a difference in the family's efforts to reach a level of adaptation as well as to assist the family member who is ill or disabled. The identification of family needs, understanding the domain of family functioning that should receive direct attention, and taking into consideration that the assistance is consistent with the family's ethnic, cultural, and religious beliefs all facilitate helping efforts. Also, providing information and support, addressing family needs, and becoming aware of personal feelings as a health provider may need attention at each period of family assistance. Of course, the type of information and quality of support may vary with each "trigger point." For example, teaching the family necessary management skills may be more appropriate during the hospital and outpatient phases and can often be enhanced by self-help groups.

At each "trigger point" the helping professional should use *connection* skills to establish a working relationship with family members. Research indicates that certain traits and characteristics of helpers appear to positively affect helping relationships (Okun, 1987). The more in touch people are with their own behaviors, feelings, and beliefs, for example, and the more able they are to communicate genuinely, clearly, and empathically their understanding of themselves to family members, the more likely they are to provide effective assistance. These *connection* skills are:

- Making families welcome
- Listening, openness, acceptance, empathy
- Soliciting family expectations

- Understanding cultural differences and respecting diversity
- Providing verbal reinforcement during family meetings

During the entire time of assisting the family, the helping professional will use different roles. These roles include assessor, provider of information, educator, developer of support systems, challenger to families, and when appropriate, advocate. Occasionally, the helper may become a facilitator of prevention, namely, offering advice to family members on the importance of being aware of escalating stressful situations. Any efforts to assist the family to detect possible problems can render the family less vulnerable to stress-induced illness or prolonged fatigue, both of which are deterrent to individual adjustment and to the development of a satisfactory or reasonable quality of life.

AN INTERVENTION APPROACH

Figure 6.1 identifies the highlights in this proposed intervention approach.

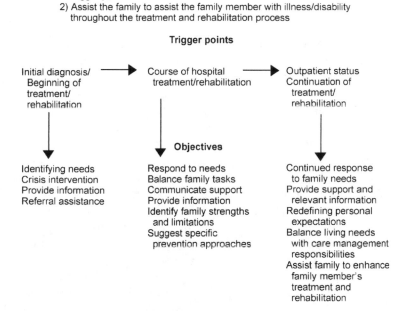

Goals: 1) Assist family members to adapt to the illness/disability at specific trigger points
2) Assist the family to assist the family member with illness/disability throughout the treatment and rehabilitation process

Trigger points

Initial diagnosis/ Beginning of treatment/ rehabilitation → Course of hospital treatment/rehabilitation → Outpatient status Continuation of treatment/ rehabilitation

Objectives

Identifying needs
Crisis intervention
Provide information
Referral assistance

Respond to needs
Balance family tasks
Communicate support
Provide information
Identify family strengths and limitations
Suggest specific prevention approaches

Continued response to family needs
Provide support and relevant information
Redefining personal expectations
Balance living needs with care management responsibilities
Assist family to enhance family member's treatment and rehabilitation

FIGURE 6.1   Proposed Intervention Approach

The proposed intervention approach emphasizes family assessment information, the setting of family meetings, and the utilization of connection skills and different helping roles. Timely assistance is based on the facts learned from a family assessment, and the priority objectives for intervention should be identified soon after this initial appraisal. From the assessment information and with input from family members, there should be agreement on the target objectives for intervention. Because of the professional's job responsibilities, the setting in which a family meeting will take place and the illness/disability related family problems that usually emerge from the medical situation, the intervention may be short-term.

Crucial to the effectiveness of any assistance are the professional's attitudes toward a particular client or family. A further discussion of these attitudes is in chapter 8. These attitudes can frequently inhibit the establishment of a working relationship with a family. Before offering any assistance to the person's family, helpers should examine their own possible prejudices, values, and limitations associated with offering support, challenging the family, and providing information and anticipatory guidance. For instance, a helper may identify with a family who needs to be temporarily taken care of and may overprotect the family or continue to protect the family when it is no longer necessary (Nelsen, 1980).

FIRST TRIGGER POINT: DIAGNOSIS/BEGINNING OF TREATMENT OR REHABILITATION

The occurrence of a disability or the diagnosis of a chronic disease is a challenging time for families. Many emotions occur among family members, such as feelings of shock, denial, anger, grief, guilt, helplessness, and intense anxiety over an uncertain future, or a very unpleasant future. Families may find it difficult to face the day-to-day consequences and implications of the disability or illness and they may not fully understand how life has really changed for them. There is the fear of losing control over the development of future plans, leaving family members with a sense of powerlessness and helplessness (Roberts, Kiselica, & Fredrickson, 2002). Also, all attention is usually on the ill family member. For many families, the onset of a disability can begin a period of intense crisis, when family members may find it difficult to meet their home and employment responsibilities, customary routines are disrupted, and the future appears uncertain. The specific objectives of intervention at this time are:

Identifying Needs: An understanding of family current and future needs at the beginning of treatment is crucial. In the authors' experience, the dominant needs of family members at this first critical point are to receive support, to have hope, be exposed to role models, to explore alternatives, and to process information. Immediately after a trauma or diagnosis, family members may need comfort more than they need information or advice. Information can come later, when it is more easily absorbed. But some families find support and comfort in the information giving process.

While the individual is undergoing critical care management in the hospital, family members usually need also to have questions answered, be reassured, and be told that someone is available to act as a resource for their own current or emerging problems. This is a very vulnerable time for the family. When assisting family members, attempts should be made to maintain a listening, nonevaluative posture that encourages the expression of feelings and questions by the family. Trust should be developed with the family, and often this can be generated by the professional's acceptance of family feelings and genuine interest in assisting family members.

Provide Crisis Intervention: If both the helping professional and family members perceive a state of crisis during this first "trigger" point, there are specific helping strategies that can be utilized. Crisis intervention with the family because of disability or illness can occur in three phases: the beginning phase, when there is the initial awareness of the trauma; the middle phase, when family members are becoming gradually or suddenly aware of the impact of the situation on both the patient and family life; and the termination phase, when family members are energetically attempting to steady the chaos caused by the crisis (Qualls, 1992). Each of these phases is relevant to varied forms of family crisis induced by the medical event. If the family's vulnerable state of equilibrium, for example, is upset by emotional outbursts, dashed expectations, or a sudden financial emergency, then there will be an initial reaction. What follows is a period when family members are aware of the impact of the crisis, and then a time when the crisis is at least temporarily resolved. Each phase, moreover, varies in length, though frequently the crisis of a severe disability or chronic illness is long term, thus creating a situation of chronic crisis and long-term need (Rolland, 1994).

Impart Information: Information that could be communicated at the beginning of treatment or rehabilitation can usually focus, when needed, on the basic facts of the illness or disability, the treatment alternatives, and the resources available to assist the family. The attending physician or nurse customarily explains the nature of the illness or disability, treatment plans, and options, but family members may not understand what is being communicated. Repetition may be necessary. Family members, because of their anxieties, are often not prepared to listen to information about the disease or disability. Also, some medical situations are not clear and the options may create more confusion and stress, e.g., lumpectomy vs. mastectomy, or surgery vs. chemotherapy or radiation. It is important, however, that confidentiality be maintained when there is an exchange of information. It is the health care professional's obligation to inform the family at the first family meeting regarding his or her policy in this regard.

Regardless of the circumstances, moreover, family members often believe that the ill member will get better. Denial operates very strongly around the time of accident occurrence and diagnosis. Though the professional may wish to provide as much information as possible about the disability or trauma, family members will usually hear what they want to hear. This is particularly true in very problematic cases where there is no cure, e.g., Alzheimer's disease or other illnesses that bring a deteriorating condition. Their initial denial of selected information may give the family time to gather emotional resources with which to deal with the implications of what has happened and what will probably happen.

Assist in Providing Referral Resources: During assessment, the professional may learn that the family appears very disturbed or quite vulnerable to a worsening of family functioning. If family members are to adjust to the demands on family life consequent to the disability or illness, then they may need help in the forms of extended, personal counseling or family therapy. The helper realizes, consequently, that his or her intervention efforts should include motivating the family to seek further professional assistance. But it may be difficult for some family members to go through with a referral. When the family is convinced that their own seeking of assistance will make a difference in their family member's treatment and rehabilitation, and they are motivated to help the patient to get better, they are often willing to obtain some needed family assistance. The helper may also share perceptions with family members, such as "I believe you are going to find that coping with this situation is very difficult, and you might need someone who can give you help for a longer period of time that I can provide."

Advising families to seek assistance for their problems is a delicate matter. It can facilitate a referral when the helper identifies and carefully explains what professional counseling or family therapy usually involves, initiates the beginning contact (such as offering to make an initial appointment with the therapist), and then later contacts the family to ascertain whether a meeting with the therapist ever took place. But the family's response to any further help may be a reflection of several factors: the relationship they are establishing with the professional, the seriousness of the patient's condition, the availability of resources, their previous exposure to role models or others who have benefited from the experience, and their own motivation to seek help for the patient's own adjustment and rehabilitation. Occasionally when the family member who is chronically ill or severely disabled is viewed by the family as responsible for the medical condition, e.g., drunk driving or carelessness with firearms, there may be ambivalent feelings about caring efforts and the member's well-being may not be a family priority.

All in all, this time of assistance is an opportunity for the professional to promote a beginning relationship with family members. A helper's awareness of the importance of good listening and showing respect for differing family viewpoints, combined with encouraging family members to express their concerns and imparting relevant information, can promote the conviction among family members that the professional is a partner in their efforts to assist the patient in reaching treatment and/ or rehabilitation goals.

SECOND TRIGGER POINT: COURSE OF HOSPITAL TREATMENT AND REHABILITATION

While the disabled or ill person is undergoing in-hospital treatment, adjustments are being made in family life to accommodate new or changing responsibilities. Family members are often trying to balance the needs of the family member living with the illness or disability with their own everyday demands of life and living. They are in the process of coming to grips with their own emotions and beginning to identify what is needed to adjust to the illness/disability experience. New considerations may also enter the family scene, such as financial issues, the necessary modification of family roles and duties, and the ever-present thought: "What is it going to be like living with our family member?" Many emotions may have subsided that arose at the occurrence of the diagnosis, such as feelings of helplessness and hopelessness, particularly as more information is gained about treatment and possible rehabilitation. But other feelings usually linger, namely, hope (realistic or not), frustration, anger, guilt, and anxiety over an uncertain future At this time of intervention the specific objectives are:

Responding to Family Needs: Certain needs may surface as the family balances the demands of the ill or disabled individual with the usual demands of a family life. These needs can be identified as: the necessity to reframe the situation in order to render it possibly less stressful; the need to marshal resources; the desire for more information on treatment and prognosis; the need to feel competent; and the growing necessity to establish a working relationship with health professionals. Communication with health professionals in a hospital setting is usually a new and frustrating experience for most family members. Their own worry over the family member's future, as well as their perception of the all-powerful role of the physicians, nurses, and other members of the health care team, so often inhibit a more initiating and assertive relationship with those responsible for the family member's care.

Attention to family needs at this time can begin with assisting family members to learn the useful skill of reframing or mentally restructuring the disability situation. Matheny, Aycock, Pugh, Curlette, and Cannella (1986) report from their extensive literature review of useful coping strategies that cognitive restructuring is the second most frequently cited coping strategy, next to relaxation exercises. A great deal of stress generated from a disability comes from stressful mental sets: from self-critical evaluations, from the fearful ballooning of potentially painful experiences, and from looking only at the worst eventualities caused by the onset of disability or illness . Other authors believe that cognitive restructuring involves engaging family members in a gentle, rational confrontation of their irrational beliefs about the disability or illness, so as to replace those beliefs with ideas that are more adaptive (Mitchell & Krumboltz, 1987). Cognitive restructuring aims, for example, to reframe the disability or illness stressor as a challenge to overcome, and attempts to place these concerns into a perspective with other life responsibilities and advantages. The helping professional can provide insights into how to identify positive outcomes inherent in living with a disabled family member. The disability, though usually causing a severe emotional impact on family members, does not have to be viewed exclusively as trouble or as a hopeless reality. This is when the exposure to role models and the life experiences of others in similar situations can be very helpful and can have a significant impact on the family . After encouraging family members to share their beliefs about what the onset of the illness or disability experience means to them, the professional can suggest that the family reflect on such ideas as: "Is it possible to identify the value to the family of what has happened?" "Is your own lot as onerous as that of others?" "Is it possible that if all of you are willing the family may grow closer because of this illness/disability?" Though it may be difficult for family members to endorse completely such ideas while the family member is still in the hospital, these suggestions may provide new perspectives on how to cope more effectively with family stressors and the emerging needs of the treatment and rehabilitation process.

The family also needs to recognize, organize, and access their personal and community resources. Because many persons tend to overlook or underestimate their coping strengths, family members need help in acknowledging these assets. Many professionals could be more effective if they directed more attention to the strengths of families. Many such strengths were identified earlier. Other resources that could be utilized by the family may include friends, support groups, and agencies that provide information on financial and legal concerns. However, many family members are often not ready during the beginning weeks of their family member's hospitalization to become involved with self-help groups. They may need time to adjust to the impact of the disability or illness. Others may be very receptive and the options related to early support should be made available.

Provide Information: As support is the primary suggested intervention for the helping professional at the time of diagnosis or trauma, so the educating of family members and the imparting of information are the most important helping efforts in the second critical period for the family. The family may further need additional, disability-related information. Earlier contacts may have been made with family members, and basic information about disability and treatment issues shared. The availability of Web sites has increased the amount of accessible information, although so much knowledge has become accessible that it may be confusing to some families to process the information and understand its impact and implications.

But some family members may still be denying the important implications of the disability for family life, such as those affecting employment or other family responsibilities. Information may then have to be provided that gradually helps the family members to face reality, keeping in mind that all members may not have the same perception of reality as the professionals on the health care team. The emphasis, though, is on *gradually,* for as stated earlier a certain amount of denial in the early stages of an illness or disability may help some family members to gain strength and support to face disability-related implications. But denial of the basic facts of the situation over an extended period of time can become destructive to both the patient and to family life, e.g., not attending to signs of cancer or heart problems by hoping they will go away. When it is appropriate, the communication of pertinent information can include highlighting the patient's residual assets and what are reasonable rehabilitation goals. Many families experience difficulties in understanding the current, in-hospital behavior of the individual, and so they tend to feel lost and frustrated. These latter difficulties may arise because of the differences in time orientation between the patient and the family. Lilliston (1985) explains that the patient's future perspective may be only as long as the next round of medication that manages pain. The patient's preoccupation with present bodily sensations and bodily functions absorb his or her total attention. The sphere of temporal focus is predominantly upon the present. Time for most patients moves painfully slowly, and they become bored, restless, and unhappy. But other family members tend to experience a more dynamic sense of time.

When the professional is aware of this disparity in time orientation, and recognizes other concerns that appear to be eroding the family's sense of competence in handling the disability or illness situation, the health provider may suggest ways that the family can be as involved as much as possible in the patient's care. The professional can also provide information that improves communicating and alleviates uncertainty, and again directs the family members' attentions to their own assets and their contributions to the patient's welfare. Also, communicating how the family can control the impact of the disability on family life may promote a sense of relief and security among family members. For example, the spouse of a newly disabled person may be quite worried about the possibility of future unemployment and what this would mean for the family's security. However, when the professional indicates different financial resources as well as possible vocational rehabilitation alternatives, then the spouse may begin to feel a little more optimistic about the family's future.

Identify Family Strengths and Limitations: The professional's attention to strengths can also assist family members to develop a sense of a newly established competence as they learn to adjust to the disability situation. Many factors contribute to a lowered sense of competence among family members: the new but complicated world of medical technology, the uncertainty over the specific prognosis of the disability, and the continued involvement in the hospital atmosphere, which can be impersonal, stressful, anxiety producing, and conducive to generating the belief that "perhaps we are different and something is wrong with us because this disability or accident occurred".

Balancing Family Tasks: A frequent problem that occurs with many families at this time of in-hospital treatment is that one family member can overextend herself or himself in providing attention to the individual, to the detriment of adequate family functioning. Other family members may feel resentful that a mother or father is spending so much time away from home. Once this is identified, the professional can briefly suggest ways to balance the needs of the hospitalized person with needs of other family members. Because resentment may be nurtured by a lack of communication, the helper may even encourage the parent or other family member to discuss his or her involvement with the others. Also, depending on how much the helping professional knows about a particular family's daily functioning, the helper may further provide ideas on how family life can be maintained as normally as possible for as long as possible, and how family members can take care of themselves while attending to their needs and those of the individual with illness/disability.

Many problems occur in family life at this time simply because family members did not ask the right questions, did not ask questions at all, or did not understand the helper's responses. The family needs to become aware that concerns should be identified and appropriate questions asked. Strategies that encourage this communication are discussed in Chapter 8.

Communicating Support: The helper's responses to family adjustment concerns are mainly through providing information that is educational. Yet support and prevention are two additional threads in this fabric of helping. Support during the patient's hospitalization can take the form of not only listening to the questions of family members, but also showing them that what they have said makes sense and has been understood. Family members will also harbor many negative feelings because of the perceived threats to family life generated by the disability situation. The professional can reassure the family that many of their negative feelings are to be expected. Allowing family members to ventilate their feelings can reassure them that the professional is supportive of their coping efforts

An issue that is frequently raised at this time is what kind of support to offer the family. As Nelsen (1980) states, most professionals will have already accepted the reality of the family situation when taking an assessment. Family members will often benefit from this accepting atmosphere and plan solutions to their problems. They may need no other type of support. Yet some families with many available resources to use in the resolution of a problem may lack confidence to take advantage of these resources. Nelsen believes that validation should be extended to the family, namely, feedback to family members using these resources that they are on the right track, that they possess personal and family strengths to cope with the situation, and that they have the confidence of the helper.

Suggested Prevention Approaches: Prevention is another form of intervention during this second critical period for family members. It implies that the professional will assist family members to recognize potential stressors and vulnerabilities and identify additional, needed resources to meet these demands. Such stressors may include a family member's prolonged absence from the home or a change in family duties and responsibilities. Both of these events may have occurred earlier in family life, but now, because of the different issues created by an illness or disability, previous coping strategies may be inadequate. In handling difficult times and situations, families frequently prefer to look to their own immediate family for any assistance. Some people, however, do not have families and others have families whom they do not want involved in the treatment and/or rehabilitation process. When the helping professional perceives, however, that a family member's absence, a change in family duties, or impending care-giving responsibilities at home may cause undue stress to family members, then the helper should encourage the use of outside resources. In fact, when there are severe financial concerns or, for instance, when a home needs architectural modifications because of the person's disability, then outside resources must be promoted, if available, to family members.

The issues of architectural redesign are troubling ones for many families. Though persons with such disabilities as quadriplegia, paraplegia, and spina bifida will usually need functional changes in the home, some parents of disabled children tend to delay making environmental adaptations. Exterior home changes (e.g., ramps or enlarged entranceways) may stimulate feelings of stigma among family members; in addition, the family may actually have difficulty accepting the implications of the disability for family life (Lewis, 1985). During the time of hospitalization and institutional, long-term rehabilitation, the family may have moved on with its routine of life and living. They have been able to visit the hospital or rehabilitation center on their own time and have, in effect, developed a built-in respite process. It may be more of a burden for the person to return home and consequently there is some hesitation from family members to disrupt or change an established pattern of living. This may conflict with the desire of the family member to get home as soon as possible.

Professionals should be aware of impending difficulties for the family member when he or she returns home, and should attempt to assist the family to prepare for the necessary changes. The helper, during family contacts, can encourage the goals of mobility, independence, and normalization for the person, urge parents to get in touch with parent groups where other parents can explain what home improvements have been made in the past and what they have learned from these adaptations, and remind family members that a delay in removing architectural barriers can frequently lead to severe stress and continued anxiety (Lewis, 1985).

During this intervention period, consequently, the helping professional continues to listen and encourages family members to understand not only the possible problem areas for adjustment, but also their own internal and external resources that can be utilized to deal with what has happened. The family is also stimulated to enter into a dialogue in which mutual feelings can be recognized and different solutions can be shared to the varied problems emerging from the medical situation. The intervention approaches of education, support, and prevention, therefore, also help the family to alleviate stress, to maintain normal patterns of living, and to become aware of their strengths and limitations. All of these strategies are beginning steps for family members that lead to their possible roles as resources for the ill person's eventual rehabilitation. The groundwork for this is developed before the family member returns home.

THIRD TRIGGER POINT: OUTPATIENT STATUS, AND CONTINUATION OF TREATMENT/REHABILITATION

This stage embraces those weeks, months, and sometimes years that the family member is recuperating at home and continuing to learn how to live with the disability or illness. It may also include that time when the chronic illness or disability has been finally stabilized, if possible, and family members are settling into the routine of living with a person with chronic illness or disability. Pollin (1995) believes that when an individual is released from a medical facility, this can be an effective time for another step in the intervention process. The extent of family contact with the health care team who provided education and support during the previous two critical points, moreover, usually diminishes over time. Many other helping professionals may now become newly involved with the family. Some of these are rehabilitation nurses, psychologists, visiting home-care nurses, medical social workers, and rehabilitation counselors.

For a family member leaving the hospital after many weeks or months of treatment, a return to the home and available family can be a turning point for his/her daily adjustment and eventual rehabilitation. Unfortunately, the home can become a refuge, a place of moratorium, where the family member who is chronically ill or disabled may fall into a comfortable routine and neglect to seek possible opportunities and renewed activities, e.g., recreation, education, or work. On the other hand, the home can become a valuable resource, where families are viewed not only as responsible, care-giving agents who provide substantial physical, emotional, and social support, but also as continued facilitators for the patient's productivity and achievement of rehabilitation goals.

Whether the family becomes an important resource, or represents a deterrent to adjustment and rehabilitation, can often be determined as the family gathers to consider or to bring their family member home, rather than to alternative living arrangements or a nursing home. Efforts should be made by the helping professional to have some family contact at this time. It is hoped that this would not be the first time that the helper has met the patient's family members. But if it is, in many hospital settings such a meeting is a structured time when information is usually provided to the family on patient needs. Discharge planning is conducted during this meeting, and preferably the patient's family has been included in the development of plans. If the discharge plan is to be realistic and viable, the provision of an aftercare plan that includes the family's recommendations, capabilities, and resources for their relative's rehabilitation and/or treatment program should be considered (McElroy, 1987).

When the family member has returned home and is undergoing treatment and/or rehabilitation on an out-patient basis, there is the particular opportunity for other available family members to become a vital resource during this period of disability or illness management. They can make a difference in how the family member responds to health care interventions. As will be discussed later in this chapter, including the individual in household tasks and social activities, providing transportation when needed to medical appointments, and urging the family member to be as active as possible, are just a few behaviors that can enhance self-esteem and make a difference in the disabled or ill person's response to treatment/rehabilitation efforts. There are also selected objectives during this third "trigger point" outlined in Figure 3 that are foundational both for the family to become a useful partner in the family member's health care, and for their own efforts to adapt to the transition of a change in family life with a return to home and entering outpatient status of the ill or disabled person.

Responding to Family Needs: Having gathered information on who will be mainly responsible for the care of the disabled or ill family member, by choice or by default, what the family's expectations are for the patient, and what emotions the family has about the person's re-entry, the professional can filter these issues into one main focus for intervention, namely, family needs. A family assessment conducted at the beginning of the family meeting can provide information on what the family actually needs at this time, and not what the professional believes the family needs. What professionals want and what families want from each other may be quite different. Spaniol, Zipple, and Fitzgerald (1985) believe that "assuming what families want without adequately checking out underlying assumptions usually leads to families discounted, devalued, and disenfranchised by professional intervention" (p. 4). The family's viewpoint on needed services is extremely important, for how well the family manages the ill family member's adjustment and rehabilitation depends on the kinds and qualities of services designed to help them (Power & Dell Orto, 1980; Power, Dell Orto, & Gibbons, 1988).

The authors have learned from family members that at the time of hospital discharge their needs are varied and often include the need to express their feelings on the patient's return home and the need for information. The latter is especially related to how they can assist the family member at home; what are effective behavioral-management techniques; where particular services can be provided; and, when possible, what is involved in the vocational rehabilitation process. Additional family needs are: knowing how to handle caregiver fatigue and possible burnout; maintaining a normal life; building a fulfilling life for themselves; sustaining a productive relationship with health professionals; and developing more personal skills of managing and parenting. The professional's response to all of these needs suggests the intervention forms of education, support, providing options, and prevention, with an emphasis on attention to the family's educational needs. Sharing of information by the professional must contain language that is easy for the family to understand. Providing information alone, however, is sometimes not enough. Though the communication of important facts about disease or disability management conveys a form of support to family members, often words of encouragement for future care giving efforts can impart reassurance.

Providing Support and Relevant Information: Allowing family members to discuss their feelings about and problems with caring for the person at home during an additional family meeting is another form of support that can be provided by the professional. When issues are raised about possible difficulties in taking care of the family member, the family may not only be seeking answers to treatment questions, but may also be looking for validation of what they propose to do for their family member. An accepting, reassuring attitude from the professional can promote feelings of confidence within the family. But this communication becomes problematic when there are major differences between the expectations of the family and those of the health care professional. When family members have more information about management concerns, moreover, the course of treatment, available resources, and the support that can be provided by helping professionals, then they frequently feel better about their home responsibilities with the individual who is disabled or ill.

One specific information area that may need to be reemphasized is what the family can do to involve the member in family life and responsibilities. Some families, however, may not wish to be involved because of the emotional and physical price to be paid. Also, though initially enthusiastic about urging this individual to be productive within the home, family members may diminish their efforts if the person wants to maintain a dependent role, or if warranted, entitlement benefits begin, or if the caregiver becomes so fatigued that only the essential treatment duties can be provided. Unfortunately, after leaving the hospital many adults with a chronic illness or disability never return to their former employment or level of productivity, even when it is possible. Although there are many reasons for this occurrence, such as employer attitudes, depression over lost capabilities, and few existing opportunities for retraining in a particular geographic area, the family should be aware that they have a definite role in their family member's rehabilitation progress. Basic to this role are the family's positive expectations within the home for the productivity of the person. The professional's viewpoints on these expectations may have to be stated again sometime during the outpatient phase.

Other facts that can be communicated during this "trigger" point are what additional community resources family members could utilize, and what happens to someone when he/she begins the process of vocational rehabilitation. Among available resources, self-help groups are particularly valuable for families after living with the individual for a few weeks, or even before the family member returns home. These groups can help the family to meet social needs, needs for hope, and be a sustaining force in the week-to-week lives of individuals who have assumed the daily burden of care (Dell Orto & Lasky, 1979; Spaniol, 1987).

Information on the vocational rehabilitation process is important to convey to family members. When this involvement is a possibility, an understanding of each step in the process can alleviate many frustrations and uncertainties. Family members are usually strangers to the services provided for people with illness and disability. They may also harbor negative attitudes or misunderstandings about these opportunities. But a detailed explanation of what is available, the time usually required to receive the service, and what may be a few of the difficulties when participating in a specific resource can alleviate many concerns and even serve as a motivating factor, when it is feasible, for one's rehabilitation. When their fears are allayed, then family members may be more willing to endorse the lengthy process of vocational rehabilitation.

During this outpatient phase of the family member's rehabilitation, however, a sudden worsening or exacerbation of the illness or disability may occur. Such an event can be predicted with certain medical conditions, e.g., multiple sclerosis, mental illness, or Alzheimer's disease. These perceived changes can represent a serious crisis for the family, and crisis-management skills may have to be utilized by the professional. Yet, when exacerbations occur or the clinical course of a disability or chronic illness is uncertain, professionals should be clear with families about the complexity of the condition and the limitations of current knowledge or treatment. Families need to hear that professionals also are struggling to determine how best to help their family member. This awareness will help families to come to terms with their own hopes, fears, and limitations (Zipple & Spaniol, 1987).

Redefining Personal Expectations: Communication of relevant information that highlights the family's role in treatment and/or rehabilitation should emphasize the family's expectations for their family member. Family members frequently encourage the individual to remain in the "sick" role. The family's almost exclusive attention to what the person cannot do, combined with the apparent availability of entitlement benefits, encourages the conviction that he/she should remain inactive at home. Expectations related to the sick role also flow from the family understanding of the disability. For example, if the family incorrectly perceives that the disability or illness causes a person to be different, rather than just to act differently on occasion, then family members place the individual in a dependent role that may be unwarranted by the condition. This attitude usually prevents the family member from returning to many family duties, and often suggests to this person that he/she should relinquish even satisfying social activities.

The helper, consequently, can assist family members to direct their attention to the person's capabilities, and to provide reinforcement for the performance of treatment duties and family responsibilities. Through all of these activities, the person with the disability can get in touch again with one's strengths. This awareness, and the accompanying feeling of competence and usefulness, may be added motivating factors to reach rehabilitation goals (Power & Dell Orto, 1980).

Balancing Living Needs with Care Management Responsibilities: An additional area of information that may need restating is how to balance care-giving responsibilities with the caregiver's personal needs. Though attention has been given at an earlier time of intervention as to how family life can be maintained as normally as possible, care-giving is a relentless, demanding task of dealing with the everyday family and treatment duties for someone with a severe disability or chronic illness. The demands on time and the energy required are often a tremendous drain on a family member's personal resources. Also, feelings of guilt and worry, or the nagging question: "What would happen if I were not there?" often inhibit someone from seeking temporary relief from the continued demands of care giving. Over a long period of time family members may realize that the disability situation is not likely to change radically for the better, and this perspective may cause families to be further drained and worn out (Spaniol, 1987). To maintain the necessary balance, a few suggestions can be offered by the professional. These include exploring meaningful work outside the home, seeking the companionship of close friends, or performing a favorite, enriching activity. These ideas may have been provided earlier in the adjustment process, but their repetition may find a more receptive audience after family members have experienced the everyday burdens of care giving. Respite care issues are discussed in Chapter 10.

During the family meetings the professional can remind family members that if they don't take good care of themselves, then they really cannot take good care of the disabled or ill family member. Families often need permission to put greater time and energy into themselves and should frequently refocus much of their energy on their own needs and wants. When the professional can suggest positive options for family members, which may include activities such as spending time alone or with old friends, going to the theater, getting away on weekends, and reinvolving themselves in activities that have nothing to do with disability and illness, then such suggestions may facilitate the belief that they can make their life work for themselves on a daily basis (Zipple & Spaniol, 1987).

Helping professionals can also indicate to the family that one way to alleviate possible fatigue is to alter stress-inducing behavior patterns in the home. In other words, family members need to adjust the demands on them to the limitations of their own resources. The goal of this strategy is to balance the demand-resource equation by advising families to become aware of escalating stress situations. Other dimensions of this strategy are to urge a family member to discuss her or his need for some free time with other family members, and remind families to be supportive of this need. It is also helpful to remind families to work toward what is possible in the situation rather than maintaining unrealistic expectations. Much family burnout is caused by the unrealistic expectations a family member holds for himself or herself.

With this attention to family-member fatigue is the accompanying emphasis on the family's need to lead a fulfilling life. But a fulfilling life develops from a family member's sense of positive self-esteem. With persons facing the severe adaptational challenges that disability and chronic illness create, self-esteem must be maintained, at all costs and enhanced, if at all possible. In other words, family members need to feel an inner assurance that they can do things necessary for a satisfactory life. Also, while living with the illness experience there may be attention to what has gone wrong in the family, thus affecting a person's self-image. An identification and appreciation of what is working well in the family may renew self-esteem (Brand, 1995). Personal worth is also reinforced by the care and concern exhibited by the professional, by a network of friends and relatives, and by an understanding of personal and family strengths. In recognizing these assets, family members can often begin to feel better about themselves and then take additional steps to pursue satisfying activities.

The threads of education, support, and prevention, consequently, form the pattern of helping at the time the patient leaves the hospital, returns home, and at family meetings during the extended treatment and rehabilitation process. The intervention through education particularly responds to the many concerns and challenges that family members will face when caring the person who is ill or disabled. But family meetings can be perceived as a mutual interaction process between family members and the helping professional. This contact is designed both to promote the person's well-being and to assist the family in their coping efforts. Developing positive expectations for the person experiencing the illness or disability, providing appropriate information to all family members, facilitating the utilization of support systems, developing family competencies, and encouraging confidence within the family in their care-giving responsibilities are each intervention objectives that can help the family member to reach an optimal level of functioning.

Assist Family to Enhance Family Member's Treatment and Rehabilitation: The available family can make a unique difference in their member's treatment and rehabilitation by playing a vital role when this individual returns home and becomes an outpatient. The family is not to become a therapeutic community, but an ongoing resource during post-hospital care management. There are several ways for family members to provide assistance during this important period for the person with a disability or chronic illness, such as:

1. *Becoming aware of what the ill or disabled person is emotionally going through upon re-entering family life after perhaps a long hospital stay.* The emotional and behavioral reactions were discussed in chapters two and three. Though there may be a sense of relief that in-hospital treatment is over, intense emotions of anger, guilt and anxiety over the future can linger. This child, teen-ager, or adult may feel vulnerable and is still attempting to deal with all the emotions associated with loss. But a family member's awareness that particular emotions could still be present, and giving the individuals a chance, if willing, to ventilate or to discuss personal feelings without a judgmental response, could gradually pave the way for both management of the emotions and a beginning step towards a form of life productivity.

2. *Involving the ill or disabled person in family household and social activities.* Often, upon discharge from the hospital, family members still place the person in a "sick role," unnecessarily protecting the individual from responsibilities and opportunities representing a gradual return, when appropriate, to pre-injury or pre-disability activities. Suggestions related to this involvement have been made earlier in this chapter. They are all directed to emphasizing what the individual can do, to one's residual or restored strengths. Encouraging usefulness in the family, and participation in family leisure and social activities can be another step towards helping this person to a productive lifestyle.

3. *Providing specific help associated with treatment and rehabilitation goals.* This assistance can include transportation, reminders of taking medication, and identifying helping opportunities that have not been part of the family's leisure activities. Alerting the family member who is coping with illness or disability adjustment demands to self-help groups or other related community activities is an example of this specific assistance.

4. *Being aware of one's attitude towards the family member who has returned to family life and now must manage the tasks of adaptation and perhaps the challenges associated with beginning a new life.* Unfinished business over incidents in family life that occurred prior to disability or illness onset, or anger and resentment caused by circumstances related to this onset, may inhibit more positive attitudes towards the family member. These positive attitudes are characterized by attention to the person's residual physical, intellectual, and emotional strengths and by the conviction that eventually the family member who is disabled or chronically ill can resume many family and even employment related activities.

The helping professional has a contribution, when appropriate, to the implementation of this second intervention goal. At an opportune time, suggestions can be made to the family on how all available family members can be instrumental in the person's treatment and rehabilitation. These suggestions may emerge from a family assessment that also highlights the identification of who are the major players within the family for care management, and the other external and internal resources accessible to the family. Negative perceptions about rehabilitation or the future productivity of the family member could be shared. Such information may flow from a trusting relationship between the family and the helping professional. This communication may establish a foundation for added intervention efforts that emphasize providing the family with a different perspective. This intervention may be quite difficult, but one that eventually can make a difference for the family member's adjustment to one's medical condition.

Though attention in this chapter has been given to individual professional and family meetings, there are other forms of family assistance that have been quite valuable for family management and adjustment concerns. Weihs, Fisher, and Baird (2002) state that psycho educational interventions are "the most common type of family-focused interventions" (p. 17). The goals of these approaches are to increase the family's knowledge of the disease or disability, and to improve their capacity for management of the medical condition. Parents and siblings of ill children, as well as caregivers and their ill or disabled adult relatives, are the usual targets for psycho educational strategies (Weihs, Fisher, & Baird, 2002). Integral to these interventions, moreover, are behavioral change modalities and coping skills strategies.

Family counseling is another intervention technique that aims to restore equilibrium to the family system. This can be encouraged by providing the family with the information and coping strategies that will assist them to manage many of the treatment demands of the individual who is ill or disabled, while at the same time helping them to deal with the impact of the medical condition on individual family members (Roberts, Kiselica, & Fredrickson, 2002). When, after meetings with the family, it becomes apparent that family counseling or family therapy would considerably improve functioning among family members in their own coping attempts, then the health professional becomes a liaison between the family and various external support systems. Issues related to assisting the family to seek family counseling or therapy were discussed earlier in this chapter.

Group counseling has also been effective as an intervention strategy, and is discussed in detail in chapter 7. McRae and Smith (1998) believe

that sharing their stories and hearing the stories of others, group partici-
pants are assisted in normalizing their feelings and restoring a sense
of coherence and continuity. In a group environment, family members
can feel that they are not alone and gain a sense of belonging.

CONCLUSION

The emphasis on education and support provided at selected times
during the family member's treatment and rehabilitation is intended
to shift, whenever possible, the family's perception that the medical
situation is a family tragedy to one that gradually comes to view what
has happened as an opportunity for a renewal in family life through
shared experiences and for transcending the constraints caused by
illness and disability. Although family members dealing with illness or
disability may not fully regain their previous quality of life, there are
intervention approaches that improve the ability to cope and facilitate
a renewed zest for life, deeper meaning, and joy (Roberts, Kiselica, &
Fredrickson, 2002). The strategies suggested in this chapter challenge
the commonly held assumption that any enjoyment of life disappears
with the onset of illness and disability. Implied also in this approach is
the further opportunity for the family to take control of much of the
delivery of needed services and to value their care-giving experience.

Whether intervention consists primarily of counseling, education, or
support, it should also enable families to attain and maintain a reasonable quality of life. At the same time, as they perform their care-giving
roles, the family acts as a resource for the potential rehabilitation,
growth, and development of the transformed family member. Intervention should be tailored to the individual needs of families and should
focus on aiding family members to bring normalcy back into their lives
as they respond to care-giving demands. Efforts to regain the balance
in family life requires a sense of competency by family members, a
consistent emotional experience for the family, and an awareness of
their own strengths, limitations, and resources.

LOUISE: THE DAY MY WORLD TURNED

Life is, or can seem to be, unfair. Though attempts are made to have
some control over what happens to us, the unexpected still occurs.
Occasionally, positive interventions can take place that may resolve
some negative outcomes of the unexpected. Colleagues, friends, and

family members can often be the source of this assistance. Their support and encouragement may make a difference between hope and discouragement. Louise's story below highlights the importance of insightful understanding to the losses incurred by this physician.

My life changed on a Saturday morning in Iowa. As a 49-year-old orthopedic surgeon, I was on my way to the hospital to see patients when suddenly the front end of my car was hit by a car going over 75 mph, driven by a young woman who had been drinking. I was in the hospital for a week recovering from broken ribs, facial injuries, and a brain injury. Once I arrived home, I had every intention of returning to my previous duties as a physician. I had worked very hard to become a doctor and establish my practice, and I had achieved this also with the awareness that there are very few women in my specialty.

When I returned to work, I knew something was wrong. I was very tired, like something was constantly running me over. I planned in a few months for full-time resumption of my duties. I had spent my whole life getting to this point of my professional career. My husband had been killed in a hunting accident four years earlier. I was now supporting my two children because they had difficulty making it on their own. I bought a farm and they lived with me to help maintain the crops and animals. My hopes were strong about returning to my medical work. I asked the plastic surgeon about one of my major mental complaints, keeping track of time, and he said that he'd seen a lot of brain-injured persons with that concern, but that usually this symptom was gone in 3 months. I thought, "Great!"

When I was working in the hospital I used to have to keep track of 15 patients as well as their specific medical issues. I realized when I started back to work that I couldn't remember patients' names. I also couldn't meet the expectations of others. At home, I tried cleaning the bathroom and doing the wash at the same time, and I just couldn't do it. I don't know why. I was realizing that a total readjustment was needed in my personal and family lives. It was like throwing the family up in the air and wherever it landed, we would have to start growing together. Fortunately, all of us in the family wanted to grow together.

I found out that I couldn't remember what I read, and if there was a distraction I couldn't apply material read in the proper sequence. Unfortunately, I discovered that since I wasn't improving in an allotted time slot, I was beginning to be considered by other doctors as a malingerer. I was caught between being labeled a malingerer, which the head of my group practice actually called me, and not wanting to operate and take care of people because I couldn't keep track of what I was doing. I even forgot what I was seeing patients for. I'd walk into a room and call the patient by name and find I had the wrong chart in my hand and was calling the person by the wrong name. I made a lot of stupid mistakes, which indicated something was not working right. I had very little motivation and no stamina. I bottomed out before I even started to work. All in all, it was dangerous for me to see patients. I received 75 percent of the audio and visual stimuli presented to me, but I processed none of it. I was also very slow in my reaction time.

As time went by, I realized it was not realistic to resume my medical practice. I believed the chances of regaining what I lost were probably not very good. I took a series of tests and the Social Security evaluators found me "totally disabled." My insurance company would not pay for several of my large medical bills during the first year after the initial trauma. I have medical insurance now, and I'm paying the premiums at a reduced rate.

I've found that most people don't understand head injuries, especially the medical profession. I look fine; I talk fine. Therefore, I should be able to act exactly as I did before the accident. But when I try to act like I used to, I fail. It's bad enough when you criticize yourself for not being as you were before the accident, but when society reinforces it, it's worse. You need a lot of support to help you through it. My intelligence isn't gone; I just can't access it. The general medical population doesn't understand mild to moderate brain injuries and the deficits that arise from them. This is very frustrating for me. It's scary that those who should have an understanding, don't.

Sometimes, I feel like going in the house, putting a paper bag over my head, and saying, "Hey, World, I want to get off." I don't mean to commit suicide, but to be a total hermit, because dealing with people is not a thing that can be regimented. I now have a lot of trouble dealing with people and I usually need to get away from them instead of seeking them out. Presently, I am going to a cognitive retraining program and working on the farm. Though I can't do anything consistently, I've realized that now, two years after the accident, I am still in the process of waking up. For example, I didn't realize for a year and a half after the accident that my house was dirty. I thought my house was immaculately clean. When I finally woke up one day and saw dirt, which had probably been there forever, I was totally amazed.

What have helped me now are many things. I really love music, movies, animals, and the theatre. Talking with groups of other head-injured people definitely helps because they understand and they'll say, "I didn't have that, but what I had was this." You realize that as a whole group, we have a problem. I realized early on that individually we all have deficits, but as a group, we are dynamite. We realize something that the general population doesn't, namely, that we all have deficits. Before you have a head injury, you don't think you have deficits. After talking, we came up collectively with a constructive way of doing things, and I've thought how wonderful it would be if hospitals could function that way.

I think I'm not ready yet for a new career. I'm still not totally awake. I can tell when I'm waking up. I just can't tell how much further I have to go. My waking up has come in stages. Yet I've always been a "can do" person, and I have to honestly face what I can't do.

DISCUSSION QUESTIONS

1. What are the losses presented by Louise?
2. Discuss Louise's statement, "I am still waking up."

3. Has peer support been helpful?
4. What intervention approaches discussed in this chapter would be relevant to assisting Louise and her family? From this information, formulate your own intervention plan for Louise and her family.
5. During the period of Louise's return to work soon after her accident, and before she realized that it was very difficult for her to accomplish her tasks within the hospital, what intervention approach would have been helpful for Louise?

SET 6: DISABILITY AND THE FAMILY: HOW WOULD YOU LIKE TO BE DISABLED OR "DIFFERENT-ABLED" LIKE ME?

PERSPECTIVE

Imagine that you are 24 years old, living in a rehabilitation facility and have been abandoned by your family. You are often told to control your anger and to get along better with your peers because you frequently become very hostile, and primarily express this during recreation periods. How should you feel? How would you feel?

EXPLORATION

The point of this exercise is to explore some issues faced by a person living with a disability and the need to appropriately express anger, frustration, distress, and unhappiness. The challenge for the helping professional is to facilitate the expression of feeling, to reduce its negative consequences, and to create viable alternatives to counterbalance an often harsh reality.

1. Discuss the need to express anger, frustration, sadness, happiness, and hope.
2. How would you react to the loss of support?
3. How would you try to get out of depression?
4. What are the implications of the loss of family for you?
5. How would a traumatic injury impact your hopes, dreams, and aspirations?
6. Would detailed and realistic information on the severity of disability of a family member be helpful or harmful to you and your family?

7. Discuss how hope can be helpful and/or harmful.
8. Would peer group counseling be helpful to you? Why? Why not?
9. What family resources do you have? Could you rely on them?
10. What would be the most difficult implications of a disability for you? For a loved one?
11. Do you believe that "miracles" are possible even when there is limited optimism regarding physical improvements?
12. How would you spend your life if your future were altered by the occurrence of a severe disability like Louise's?
13. What would you do if your doctor told you to accept your injury in peace rather than seek out alternative treatment or experimental drugs to "cure" your illness or disability?
14. How could your family be more helpful?
15. What do you feel you would need the most if you had a severe brain injury? Cancer? A stroke?

REFERENCES

Brand, P. (1995). Coping with a chronic disease: The role of mind and spirit. *Patient Education and Counseling, 26,* 107–112.

Cohen, M. S. (1999). Families coping with childhood chronic illness: A research review. *Family Systems and Health, 17*(2), 149–163.

Dell Orto, A.E., Lasky, R. (Eds.),(1979). *Group counseling and physical disability.* Boston, MA: Duxbury Press.

Lewis, B. E. (1985). *Inventors, explorers, experimenters: How parents adapt homes for children with mobility problems.* Unpublished manuscript. West Newton, MA: Humanized Environments.

Lilliston, B. A. (1985). Psychosocial responses to traumatic physical disability. *Social Work in Health Care,* 1–7.

MacFarlene, M. (1991). Treating brain-injured clients and their families. *Family Therapy, 26,* 13–30.

McRae, C., & Smith, C. H. (1998). Chronic illness: Promoting the adjustment process. In S. Roth-Roemer, S. R. Kurpius, & C. Carmin (Eds.), *The emerging role of counseling psychology in health care.* New York: Norton.

Matheny, K. B., Aycock, D. W., Pugh, J. L., Curlette, W. L., & Cannella, K. A. (1986). Stress coping: A qualitative and quantitative synthesis with implications for treatment. *The Counseling Psychologist, 14,* 499–549.

McElroy, E. M. (1987). The beat of a different drummer. In A. Hatfield & H. Lefley (Eds.), *Families of the mentally ill.* New York: Guilford Press.

Mitchell, L. K., & Krumboltz, J. D. (1987). The effects of cognitive restructuring and decision-making training on career indecision. *Journal of Counseling Development, 66,* 171–174.

Nelsen, J. C. (1980). Support: A necessary condition for change. *Social Work,* September, 388–392.

Okun, B. E. (1987). *Effective helping: Interviewing and counseling techniques.* Monterey, CA: Brooks/Cole.

Oliver, M., & Sapey, B. (1999). *Social work with disabled people,* 2nd ed., Basingstoke: UK: Macmillan Publishers.

Pieper, B., & Singer, G. (1991). *Model family professional partnerships for interventions in children with traumatic brain injury.* Albany, NY: New York State Head Injury Association.

Pollin, I. (1995). *Medical crisis counseling: Short-term therapy for long-term illness.* New York: Norton.

Power, P. W., & Dell Orto, A. E. (1980). *Role of the family in the rehabilitation of the physically disabled.* Austin, TX: Pro-Ed Publishers.

Power, P. W., Dell Orto, A. E., & Gibbons, M. B. (1988). *Family interventions throughout chronic illness and disability.* New York: Springer Publishing.

Priestley, M. (1999). *Disability politics and community care.* London: Jessica Kingsley.

Qualls, S. H. (1992). Clinical interventions research with older families: Review and recommendations. Paper presented at the annual meeting of the Gerontological Society of America, Washington, D.C.

Roberts, S. A., Kiselica, M. S., & Fredrickson, S. A. (2002). Quality of life of persons with medical illnesses: Counseling's holistic contribution. *Journal of Counseling & Development, 80,* 422–432.

Rolland, J. S. (1994). *Families, illness, and disability.* New York: Basic Books.

Spaniol, L., Zipple, A. M., & Fitzgerald, S. (1985). How professionals can share power with families: A practical approach to working with families of the mentally ill. *Psychosocial Rehabilitation Journal, 8,* 77–84.

Spaniol, L. (1987). Coping strategies of family caregivers. In A.B. Hatfield & H. Lefley (Eds.), *Families of the mentally ill: Coping and adaptation.* New York: Guilford Press.

Swain, J., & French, S. (2000). Towards an affirmation model of disability. *Disability & Society, 15*(4), 569–582.

Weihs, K., Fisher, L., & Baird, M. (2002). Families, health, and behavior. *Family Systems and Health, 20*(1), 7–46.

Zipple, A. ,M. & Spaniol, L. (1987). Current educational and supportive models. In A. Hatfield & H. Lefley (Eds.), *Families of the mentally ill.* New York: Guilford Press.

7

Group Counseling: A Resource For Families Living With Illness or Disability

GROUPS, ILLNESS, AND DISABILITY

Group counseling can help families to cope with the challenges and demands of adapting to change and loss consequent to illness and disability. The power and potential of group counseling is that it is a means to bring people together at a time of mutual need. They have an opportunity, consequently, to share their experiences, address familial concerns, develop mutual resources, learn from each other's experiences, and explore their hopes, dreams, and aspirations. Group counseling also helps to establish a structure and common ground for the rigors and demands of the treatment and rehabilitation process (Santelli, Turnbull, & Higgins, 1999; Hibbard, et al., 2002; Pickett-Schenk, 2002; Becker-Cottrill, McFarland, & Anderson, 2003; Hecht, et al., 2003; Tomasulo, 2002; Koppelman & Bourjolly, 2001; Powell, Yeaton, Hill, & Silk 2001; Tang, 2001; Dyck, et al., 2000; Jones, Brazel, Peskind, Morelli, & Raskind, 2000).

As a result of the contributions and potential of group work with families and individuals, groups are becoming more of an integral part of the treatment and rehabilitation process (Brown, et al. , 1999; Harper, Groves, Gilliam, & Armstrong, 1999; Jaffe, 1999; Koppelman, & Bourjolly, 2001; McNulty, 2002; Lee, Cohen, Hadley, & Goodwin, 1999; Wamboldt & Levin,1995).

When group counseling is applied to family treatment and rehabilitation, it can become a counterforce to the helplessness, isolation, and

---

*Some of the material in this chapter is updated and modified from Dell Orto & Power, 2000. Reprinted with permission.

desperation families may experience during this time of major life transitions and change.

Rocchio (1998) addressed the value of family groups when she stated:

> Families find groups very helpful in gaining insight into the long-term conse-quences of brain injury, ways to recognize problems in advance of their becoming difficult issues, and sharing practical management strategies with other families (p. 16).

A major contribution of group counseling, especially when applied to illness and disability, is that it provides an opportunity for people to explore the dimensions of their common as well as unique experiences and needs while developing skills to maximize their resources through a peer-oriented and goal-oriented support system.

The appeal and relevance of group counseling to both consumers and providers of treatment and rehabilitation services are that group approaches:

1. Help place illness and disability into a life and living perspective
2. Facilitate the development of and access to resources
3. Support both the client, caregivers, and family during the process of treatment and rehabilitation
4. Expose individuals and families to role models
5. Teach the necessary skills to effectively respond to past, present, and future concerns (Dell Orto & Power, 2000)

One of the most powerful insights that can take place in a group is the awareness that group members share some common ground, resources, and potential support. Rosenthal (1987) stated:

> "Groups offer opportunities to share common experiences, problems, and solutions; vent frustration and anger; and provide emotional support. Often, family members obtain specific information about community-based re-sources that can aid their relative" (p. 56).

In addressing the potential of groups as a means to respond to isolation and alienation Cicerone, Fraser, and Clemmons (1997) commented:

> Group therapy provides a means to place the client in social situations, and therefore more closely approximate the demands of real life. This can serve to reduce the client's social isolation, and at the same time demands a broader repertoire of social and interpersonal behaviors (p. 36).

Consequently groups are a means to facilitate connectedness, reduce isolation and prepare individuals and families for the demands and rigors of the treatment and rehabilitation process.

TREATMENT AND REHABILITATION

When group work is integrated into the treatment and rehabilitation process, it provides the structure and opportunity to:

1. Expose families coping with illness and disability to role models who were able or are trying to meet the life and living challenges posed by the illness and disability of a family member
2. Provide a support system that will respond to the evolving and changing long-term needs throughout the illness and disability experience rather than be limited to the concerns associated only with acute care
3. Create a structure within which family members can respond to their individual and collective needs and receive support, understanding, and encouragement from persons in similar as well as dissimilar situations
4. Introduce family members to supports and other resources based upon the knowledge and expertise of other group members, avoiding the unnecessary strain and stress of individual families having to struggle for information that is already available
5. Teach families, when appropriate, how to cope by developing proactive rather than a reactive response to problems that are common to life and living after illness and disability
6. Provide a structure for the introduction of medical information and resources that are relevant and helpful to group members
7. Establish a consumer perspective that facilitates dialogue with the health care team with an emphasis on collaborative care
8. Create a level of accountability for all who are involved in the treatment of persons with illness and disability (a collective of families and significant others is often more aware of what should be happening compared with an individual family in a state of crisis)
9. Diffuse problems before they become overwhelming to the family or its individual members by exposing families to the problems and solutions employed by other group members

10. Enable families to share the common burden of illness and disability rather than be fragmented by the desperation that is often a by-product of isolation

11. Personalize the treatment by processing information in a caring, structured manner

12. Develop referral resources that can result in professional, personal, and social contacts, which are essential to cope with illness and disability over an extended period of time

13. Understand that the existence of a group counseling program does not mean that all problems related to illness and disability can be solved, but that critical elements in the illness and disability experience will have a better chance of receiving attention

14. Advocate for what should be offered, rather than accept what is offered, as a result of resource depletion consequent to managed care and managed cost

SELECTED CRITICAL ISSUES

In a group counseling setting, members have the opportunity to participate in an unfolding process that addresses many other issues of current and future importance. A group process that addresses the critical issues often encountered by families living with illness and disability enables the group members to confront their unique and common reality, begin to adjust to their losses, explore their options, put in place the behaviors that will enhance the conditions for stabilization, gain, and hope, and enhance the quality of life. In a sense, it is an opportunity to interact and share with people faced with similar life transitions who are coping and managing their lives, as well as learn from those who may not be as successful in coping and other life domains.

Families who are coping with the illness and disability must also address many other issues that can intensify the effects and implications of the illness and disability experience as well as deplete or stress family resources. Some of these issues are as follows:

1. Marital relationships can begin to deteriorate, and spouses may see separation, resignation, or divorce as the only way to remove and save themselves from a situation they cannot handle physically and/or emotionally. As one person stated: "I did not plan on being married to an invalid. This is far more than I bargained for. I must get out of this situation even if it means running away." In a group setting members

often can express their feelings and explore how others have addressed or handled marital issues.

2. Siblings may react in negative or positive ways as a result of the changes in the family and they may experience resentment, jealousy, parental pressure, overprotection, or disinterest. For children in a group of peers, they may be more receptive to the perspectives of others and realize that others who are in similar situations may be a source of support.

3. Substance and or alcohol abuse by a family member may develop or intensify as a means to cope with the stress, changes and losses associated with the illness/disability experience. A group member stated: "The only way I can survive is by drinking. What else do I have? I know this is only resulting in more problems and I better call AA." In a group the issues of self-defeating behaviors can be identified and addressed and group members can be encouraged and supported in their efforts to engage in more positive coping behaviors.

4. Work performance of the family member living with an illness or disability, or other family members and caregivers, may deteriorate and result in loss of job or a compromising of work performance. Groups can address the themes of work and alert members to the fact that under stress, job and work behaviors can be affected.

5. By not tending to individual or mutual needs, individual family members as well as the family as a whole can neglect themselves both physically and emotionally (Tomasulo, 2002). In a group the importance of taking care of oneself and others can not only be verbalized but group members can hear and often observe what happens if group members neglect themselves.

6. Financial pressures can be seen as a cause of disharmony when, in fact, they may be symptomatic of underlying stress that is more difficult to concretize. DeJong, Batavia, and Williams (1990) stated:

> The costs of medical care, personal care, supervision, residential care and respite care for a person with a brain injury can quickly exhaust the financial capacities of even the most prosperous families (p. 13).

Through treatment and rehabilitation groups, members have the unique opportunity of learning how others have handled financial pressures, as well as how to access resources that may help reduce the financial pressures.

7. Traditional support systems such as friends, peers, and relatives may remove themselves from supporting roles because of their inability

to respond to the emotional demands made upon them (Pickett-Schenk, 2002). One group member stated: "My family was always there for the good times, now they are nowhere to be found. Every time I call they tell me they are too upset to see my husband!" During the treatment and rehabilitation process group members often replace the family supports that have been lost. For some group members the group may be the only support system they have.

8.   Educational goals and career opportunities may be altered, changed, or lost. This is especially so for caregivers who are often faced with meeting the needs of others rather than attending to their own. Expressing the loss of her career a group member stated: "I gave up medical school to take care of my parents, and my sisters do not get what a sacrifice that was. Now they do not want me to live with them when I am recovering from surgery. I am treated better by my friends who at least offered to help out." During the group process members can be exposed to others who have created options that meet their current needs as well as address what may be possible in the future.

9.   Some families may manage well in the short term but have major problems over time. One caregiver stated: "The first year after her stroke I did very well. Now I can see that there are many new issues I did not consider. This is going to be a very long process." The group process can alert, as well as prepare, members for the skills that are required for both the present as well as the future. It may be helpful for group members to hear from others how they have coped and what they would have done differently. Critical to the group process is the role and function of group leaders as well as their skills and perspectives.

GROUP LEADERSHIP: ISSUES AND SKILLS

The group leader is more than a facilitator. He or she is in a very special role that has major impact on the overall group process, as well as the lives of the group members and their family. To function in this demanding role the leader must have skills to perform a variety of tasks.

Corey (2000) presents an overview of some tasks that he considers essential for successful overall group leadership. They are summarized as follows:

- Group leaders initiate and promote interaction by the way they structure the group and model behaviors.
- Group leaders have the task of orienting members to the group process.

- Group leaders must be capable of sensitive, active listening.
- Group leaders are responsible for creating a climate conducive to exploring personally significant issues.
- Group leaders are responsible for setting limits helping establish group rules and protecting members.
- Group leaders need to direct attention to ways in which people can profit as much as possible from the group experience (p. 451).

CHARACTERISTICS, SKILLS, AND PERSPECTIVES

Working with families living with illness and disability requires additional characteristics, skills, and perspectives (Corey, 2000; Gladding, 2003; Kline, 2003). The following is a list of some of the additional characteristics, skills, and perspectives that can be helpful to the role and functioning of a leader in groups addressing illness and disability as well as loss and change:

1. Humaneness—an appreciation of the plight, struggle, needs, fears, nightmares, hopes, and dreams of families and individuals, and which manifests itself in a caring kind, empathetic, and helpful manner.
2. Compassion—the ability to feel in a constructive and helpful way.
3. Resiliency—the ability to continue with the tasks of one's role in spite of personal emotional drain that often accompanies a repetition of "failure" or "no gain" experiences or personal losses, which may be part of the treatment and rehabilitation process.
4. Intervention skills—ability to design and implement programs and responses that are timely, creative, visionary, and relevant to the evolving and changing needs of the person and family consequent to illness and disability, as well as in other domains.
5. Medical knowledge—the ability to comprehend and present the uniqueness and complexities of an illness and disability experience, as well as the secondary conditions, distractions, and stressors that can impact on the patient, the family, and the group process.
6. Communication skills—the ability to relate to, and connect with, the person, the family, significant others, and members of the interdisciplinary health care team.
7. Ability to differentiate between individual and family problems.

8. Awareness of the energizing or synergistic effects illness and disability and other situations can have on the group process, the individual, and the family system.
9. Ability to orchestrate group process with complex and shifting themes, e.g., other life losses including illness and disability of significant others.
10. Awareness of the independent and conjoint functioning of family subsystems.
11. Ability to think and act actively rather than only reactively.
12. Ability to work with a co-leader, as well as consumers, who can be helpful with large groups and provide a mutual feedback and support system.
13. Ability to resolve personal, cultural, and ethnic prejudices related to appreciating the potential and liabilities of clients and their family members.
14. Cognitive and experiential awareness of illness and disability, as well as their consequences. Group leaders should have experienced a training format that focuses on what illness and disability mean to the person and the family. The ideal is to have a co-leader who has personally experienced the reality of an illness or disability within their family. Rolland (1994) stated that as a person and a physician he had a better understanding of the impact of illness on the family after his mother had a stroke and his wife had terminal cancer. However, personal experience alone is not adequate, just as a professional degree does not always equate with effectiveness.
15. Comprehensive understanding of models and approaches that are relevant, applicable, and useful to families challenged by an illness or disability and who are often engaged in a lifelong journey and not just a short-term destination.
16. Understanding and appreciation of the intergenerational impact of loss, illness, and disability, and how these can influence family functioning.
17. Willingness to learn from group members and appreciate their perspectives. (Dell Orto & Power, 2000, p. 106)

In addition to these skills and perspectives, it is helpful if group leaders have a broad perspective on life and living and have the ability to cognitively and experientially appreciate the impact of illness and disability, loss, and trauma on the person and on the family. In addition to the need for skills to better provide for others, professional caregivers must be aware of and attend to the need for peer support to avoid and/or cope with caregiver fatigue syndrome (Tomasulo, 2002). Given the demands of the health care environment today and the reduction in staff and resources, staff may be asked to do more, and in the process they may not attend to themselves and their needs. In these situations, peer support can be extremely helpful.

While group leaders should have at their command a variety of skills, resources, and perspectives, a group model can be more responsive to the complex needs of the treatment and rehabilitation process, especially if it is comprehensive, active, and multidimensional.

SELECTED GROUP MODELS

In reference to the application of multifamily psychoeducation groups for medically ill children and adolescents, Wamboldt & Levin (1995) presented several intervention models that include: group therapy, community support, self-help groups, education, and family therapy. While these models can be integrated into a variety of settings and address a variety of issues there is the ongoing consideration of available resources to support this application. It is important to address the fact that the more sophisticated and comprehensive a model is, the more it may require in terms of personnel and financial resources, which may, in fact, limit the appeal and adaptation of group programs in many settings. This happens when programs seek to implement groups to save money and resources, rather thanexpend them.

A relevant group counseling model must go beyond a token response to the current and emerging needs of families and individuals living the illness and disability experience. This happens when a group counseling program addresses the issues encountered and anticipated during the treatment and rehabilitation process. From the authors' perspective the following are some of the selected characteristics of a multidimensional treatment and rehabilitation group counseling model that may be of help to families:

1. Is available throughout the illness disability experience
2. Has the potential to be adapted to a variety of settings (e.g., community, home, hospital, independent living, or rehabilitation facility)
3. Is flexible in meeting the evolving and changing needs of the person and the family
4. Can be fully integrated into a treatment and rehabilitation program, and has the emotional and financial support of administration and staff

5. Is capable of transcending the hospital environment and meeting the demands faced by the person and family living or attempting to live in the community
6. Has didactic components to teach the skills needed to respond to a range of medical and nonmedical problems related to the illness and disability
7. Can respond to other life losses, e.g., secondary conditions that may play an important role in adjustment to the illness or disability experience
8. Is capable of anticipating problems rather than just reacting to them (Dell Orto & Power, 2000, p. 107)

With a multidimensional group model, the needs of the families can be better met by providing a system of alternatives as well as supplementary groups which emerge from and are related to a primary family group. The family group is often the core group focusing on family issues. It is from this group that the other groups may evolve and can be connected.

The following is a list of some additional potential supplementary groups and their focus:

- Peer group—focuses on needs of the person in a group of peers
- Female group—addresses role issues which are relative to female issues and concerns
- Male group—addresses role issues that are relative to male issues and concerns. These could include cross cultural and psychosocial adjustment considerations. (Marini, 2001)
- Children/sibling group—opportunity for children to share feelings and learn how to respond to their unique situations (e.g., the injury of a parent or the stress related to a sibling undergoing aggressive treatment). Wamboldt & Levin (1995) indicated that siblings have a difficult time in verbalizing and expressing their concerns.
- Spouse/marital group—concerned with nurturing and maintaining a realistic marital relationship while coping with a traumatic injury, the importance of which is stated, for example by Zeigler (1989):

Spouses of brain injury survivors face particular problems, which are often not addressed in brain-injury family support groups. These issues can be effectively dealt with in mutual support groups. Since the number of spouses affected by brain injury is less than the number of parents who are affected, the availability of spouse support groups is limited. (p. 37)

- Caregiver and significant others group—an opportunity to involve those persons who are a part of the families' or clients' support system (Jacobs, 1997)
- Didactic group—provides information and teaches relevant skills related to living in with an illness or disability (Wiseman-Hanks, et al., 1998)
- Theme group—permits the addressing of various issues related to the illness or disability experience, e.g., parenting, independent living, wellness, sexuality, substance abuse, etc.
- Medical staff group—opportunity for health workers to discuss issues related to their individual functioning and to provide mutual support
- Educational and vocational rehabilitation group—addressing issues related to education, employment, and careers
- Life and living group—focusing on the process of developing a quality of life and living in spite of, and in concert with, an illness or disability; focus can be on what is left rather than on what was lost (Dell Orto & Power, 2000)

It is important to recognize however, that group counseling is not a magic solution to all the problems, concerns, and needs of people and families living with illness and disability. For some individuals and families the group process may not be appropriate due to the nature and complexity of their limitations or their unique circumstances. In such situations, the criteria for group intervention must be whether or not a group will contribute positively to the family's life and living experience. Also, it is important to note that some of the motivation to initiate group counseling may be motivated primarily by financial concerns, e.g., being able to provide more services with fewer staff. This is an important point to consider when, for some health care delivery systems, the needs of the patients are often beyond the allocated or accessible resources and groups may be seen as a quick fix rather than as an important component of a comprehensive service delivery system.

CONCLUSION

Group counseling with families and individuals challenged by and living with illness and disability is a major resource in personalizing the health care, treatment, research, and rehabilitation process. When relating the application of group counseling to families living with a chronic illness, it is important to address and understand the family's very individualized experiences. These are not only the general issues of life and living but also past experiences of working with other people and sharing very personal experiences and emotions. For some families and in some cultures discussing such experiences and feelings may be limited and may not be approved. This may be a due in part to the belief that only the family can be relied on and that it is not appropriate to share feeling, needs, or issues with "strangers" or others who are not members of the family. This may extend beyond the group and could relate even to the health care team.

Group counseling is also a vehicle for potential support, mutuality, sensitivity, honesty, caring, concern, and consistency, all of which can facilitate the adjustment to living with the effects and realities associated with an illness or disability.

JAMES: MY GROUP JOURNEY, WITH THE HELP OF MY FRIENDS

A major contribution of group counseling is that people can share their pain, sorrow, success, joy, and hope, while realizing that they are not alone. Frequently they are traveling a road that has been traveled before and can gain from the experiences and perspectives of others. The following personal statement focuses on the experience of being a group member in a rehabilitation hospital.

> I knew that I was in trouble when I woke up. I really did think that it was all a dream, or better yet, a nightmare. The sounds, the noise, the lights, and the surreal nature of slipping in and out of awareness. I thought that people were there, I saw their faces and heard their voices, but when I tried to reach out I was alone.
>
> This sense of isolation and fear was part of my every day experience until I realized that this was for real and that I was in big trouble. I could not move and I had a lot of alien things, tubes and monitors, attached to me. My first response was to jump out of the window. Great idea, but I could not get my self out of bed to do it. The irony is that my room was on the ground floor! Day by day I became more angry and enraged, not so much because of my injury but more so because of the circumstances, which were that I was pushed off a balcony while fighting with a friend. We were both drunk and were fighting because we wanted to date the same girl and neither of us realized that she was married. What a crazy situation! Now I am a cripple, in effect, over a very stupid situation.
>
> In addition I felt nothing was right. My family did not come to see me and, in effect, I was glad that they did not. It was just too painful for all of us, and in reality I was in such bad emotional shape that I did not blame

anyone for not wanting to be around me. I was at the end of my rope, and I think that the staff was also fed up with me and on occasion they let me know.

The situation began to change when a nurse who was one of the "good guys" (meaning that she had a smile and was very nice) mentioned that it may be helpful for me to go to a group and to meet some people who were in the same, similar, or even worse situation than I was. I rejected the idea for weeks 'til one day when I opened my eyes and at the end of my bed was a young woman in a power chair who by all appearances looked far worse off than I felt. With a smile she said he wanted to invite me to coffee in the cafeteria and I, for some reason, said "yes" even though it involved a big production to get me there. I think it was also because I was very desperate and my rage, anger, and isolation was not getting me anywhere. Also, I did not have a girlfriend and I did enjoy the company of girls. While this was not ideal (she was not very good looking but neither am I), it was certainly better than nothing, and more importantly she appeared to be a very nice person with a great spirit that transcended her physical condition.

When we talked I realized that my new friend had a lot more going for her than I did. She was upbeat, enjoyed being alive a lot more than I did, and was from all appearances in a much better place than I was. Not only did I admire her, I greatly respected her and appreciated the fact that she reached out to me. I know that at that point in time, if the shoe was on the other foot, I would not have reached out to her. When I asked her how she copes, she told me that she felt as I did about a year ago when she was in a car accident. In reality, it was a truck that ran over her car when the driver who was drunk crossed the divider and killed her parents and sisters. At the time she told me that she felt her world had ended and she did not want to live and felt she just could not go on. She told me the difference for her was that she joined a group in the rehabilitation center. As a result she had the chance to meet and connect with other people who were both better and worse off than she was. She also said that she realized that there were many others in the groups that she had participated in who would give anything to be as far along as she was and to be able to enjoy the quality of life that she had even though she has many losses in her life. This was most interesting because until that point in time she told me that she felt that her life was over and that she did not want to live as she was and without her family. For her this began to change when she took advantage of the group and used it to create a new perspective. When I heard this I felt that I had nothing to lose and out of respect for what she had been though and her efforts to reach out to me, I joined the group.

My initial response was one of relief as well as fear. The group leaders, a social worker and a nurse, were warm and welcoming. My fear was focused on the members who I knew could challenge me and force me to look at who I was and was becoming. In effect I had to rely on them and sort out what was helpful and or not relevant. When I said I would walk again, they said "maybe." When I said I could not go on they said they understood but would like me to hang in there. As I reflect on the seven months, I must say that the group counseling helped me to sort out what had happened to me and what I could expect and work for. It was different from talking to a psychiatrist or psychologist. They were helpful but in a different way. The group became my in-hospital family. They were always there, which sometimes was a problem because some members wanted to hang out with me all the time and I preferred being alone or with some of my good friends. This made me feel bad because there were people just as desperate as I was and they were looking to me to help support them. After a lot of soul searching I realized that the shoe could be on the other foot and I made an effort to be as supportive as I could and to think of the others, not just focus on my self. This was a breakthrough.

The other issue that impacted me was that some group members were able to move on and do well, while others deteriorated and a few died. The deaths were very hard on me especially when a 19-year-old group member whose world changed when he was a bystander during a robbery and was shot by accident. As he said, "wrong place, wrong time." A few days before he died, he told me, "hang in there and do something with your life." He told me he has a lot he wanted to do in his life, e.g., go to Europe, get a sailboat, and own a horse, and he hoped that I would take advantage of all I had to look forward to. His last words to me were "I wish I was as lucky as you and could do all that you can." This stopped me cold and made me think a lot. It was a major turning point for me to look at what I could do and realize that this young man would not have the opportunity to fulfill his dreams. It was a very sobering moment in my life.

My next big step was to begin to be responsive to the efforts of my family and for all of us to become part of a family group. While this was helpful to a degree, I felt that meeting only once a month was not often enough. I am not sure that my parents and sister felt this way because it was a three-hour drive, so more often may have been a problem. What I did value was the fact that my family did come and did get to meet other families who, like their family member in the hospital, were better or worse off than we were. Some had other ill or sick family members, others had very bad relationships, some were rich, others poor, but they all had something to contribute and to say. This was very helpful because I saw my friends and the other group members in the context of their family and could better appreciate what they were talking or complaining about.

My life is much better than it was. This is a result of a lot of support and the hard work that I did. I also feel that the group was a big help to me. To all of my group member friends, Thank you for tolerating me and helping me move out of the abyss of darkness!

DISCUSSION QUESTIONS

1. What is your initial response to this personal statement? Do you have any ideas what could have been helpful to this person?
2. Is it helpful to have group members being exposed to situations that are much worse or much better than their own?

3. Discuss how the circumstances related to the onset of an illness or disability can help or impede family and personal adjustment.
4. In this case, when should the family have access to a family support group?
5. Do you think that family groups should be limited only to individuals who have spouses or children who are living with a disability?
6. What are some advantages and disadvantages of having mixed groups?
7. How long do you think a support group should be made available to people with disabilities and their families?
8. What are the advantages and disadvantages of group leaders not experiencing serious illness and trauma?

SET 7: COMMON PAIN, MUTUAL SUPPORT

PERSPECTIVE

As a direct or indirect consequence of illness and disability, some individuals and families are often abandoned, isolated, and left on their own. Group counseling can provide a helpful alternative for families challenged by illness or disability by providing structure, support, and resources at a time of ongoing crisis, as well as a counterbalance to the loss of support. When thinking about group counseling and self-help alternatives, it is important to recognize that some families are not accustomed to sharing feelings with strangers and may resist the group counseling experience. In such cases, gradual exposure to group members may create the needed bridges to help families find a common ground and become receptive to a group experience.

EXPLORATION

1. Discuss how group counseling could help you and your family adjust to living with the effects of an illness or disability?
2. If you had an illness and/or disability, would you voluntarily enter a group? Why or why not?
3. What would be the most difficult aspect of group counseling for you as a group member?
4. What would be the most difficult aspect for you as a group leader?

5. Are there certain people with illnesses or disabilities you would not want to associate with?
6. List the characteristics of group members that make you uncomfortable. What are the characteristics of a group leader that would put you off?
7. Should people with and without disabilities be in the same group? Why or why not?
8. What are the advantages and disadvantages of having families coping with illness such as stroke, cancer, AIDS, etc., participate in the same group as families affected by other conditions?
9. What are the advantages and disadvantages of "professionally" led groups and groups led by survivors?
10. From your perspective, what is and should be the primary goal of group counseling for families who have experienced an illness or disability?
11. Should the person with an illness and/or disability always be part of the family group?
12. What are the disadvantages and limitations of a group counseling program for families living with an illness and or disability?
13. At what point during treatment and rehabilitation should family members join a group?
14. Identify and discuss some reasonable expectations that family members may have of the group process.

REFERENCES

Becker-Cottrill, B., McFarland, J., & Anderson,V. (2003). A model of positive behavioral support for individuals with autism and their families: The family focus process. *Focus on Autism and other Developmental Disabilities, 18*(2), 113–123.

Brown, R., Pain, K., Berwald, C., Hirschi, P., Delhanty, R., & Miller, H. (1999). Distant education and caregiver support groups: Comparison of traditional and telephone groups. *Journal of Head Trauma Rehabilitation, 14*(3), 257–268.

Cicerone, K. D., Fraser, R., & Clemmons, D. (1997). *Counseling interactions with traumatically brain injured clients.* Boca Raton, FL: CRC Press.

Corey, G. (2000). *The theory and practice of group counseling,* 5th ed. Belmont, CA: Brooks Cole.

DeJong, G., Batavia, A. I., & Williams, J. M. (1990). Who is responsible for the lifelong well being of a person with a brain injury? *Journal of Head Trauma and Rehabilitation, 5*(1), 9–22.

Dell Orto, A. E., & Power, P. W. (2000). *Brain injury and the family: A life and living perspective,* Boca Raton, FL: CRC Press.

Dyck, D. G., Short, R. A., Hendryx, M. S., Norell, D., Myers, M., Patterson, T., McDonell, M. G., Voss, W. D., & McFarlane, W. R. (2000). Management of negative symptoms among patients with schizophrenia attending multiple-family groups. *Psychiatric Services, 51*(4), 513–519.

Gladding, S. (2003). *Group work: A counseling specialty,* 4th ed. Upper Saddle River, NJ: Merrill-Prentice Hall.

Harper, W., Groves, J., Gilliam, J., & Armstrong, C. (1999). Rethinking the place of psychological support groups in cardiopulmonary rehabilitation. *Journal of Cardiopulmonary Rehabilitation, 19*(1), 18–21.

Hibbard, M., Cantor, J., Charatz, H., Rosenthal, R. I., & Ashman, T. (2002). Peer support in the community: Initial findings of a mentoring program for individuals with traumatic brain injury and their families. *Journal of Head Trauma Rehabilitation, 17*(2), 112–131.

Hecht, M. J., Graesel, E., Tigges, S., Hillemacher, T., Winterholler, M., Hilz, M. J., Heuss, D., & Neundo, B. (2003). Burden of care in amyotrophic lateral sclerosis. *Palliative Medicine, 17,* 327–333.

Jacobs, H. E. (1997). In sickness and health: At the caregiver support group. *Family Systems & Health, 15,* 213–222.

Jaffe, M. S. (1999). Support group for adults with cortical visual impairment: An innovative model. *Journal of Visual Impairment and Blindness, 93*(11), 728–732.

Jones, L., Brazel, D., Peskind, E. R., Morelli, T., & Raskind, M. A. (2000). Group therapy program for African-American veterans with posttraumatic stress disorder. *Psychiatric Services, 51*(9), 1177–1179.

Kline, W. B. (2003). *Interactive group counseling and therapy.* Upper Saddle River, NJ: Merrill-Prentice Hall.

Koppelman, N. F., & Bourjolly, J. N. (2001). Conducting focus groups with women with severe psychiatric disabilities: A methodological overview. *Psychiatric Rehabilitation Journal, 25*(2), 142–151.

Lee, M. R., Cohen, L., Hadley, S. W., & Goodwin, F. K. (1999). Cognitive-behavioral group therapy with medication for depressed gay men with AIDS or symptomatic HIV infection. *Psychiatric Services, 50*(7–, 948-952.

Marini, I. (2001). Cross cultural counseling with males who sustain a disability. *Journal of Applied Rehabilitation Counseling, 32*(1), 36–44.

McNulty, K. (2002). Psychological and emotional recovery to severe burn injury. *Journal of Applied Rehabilitation Counseling, 33*(1), 7–12.

Pickett-Schenk, S. A. (2002). Church-based support groups for African American families coping with mental illness: Outreach and outcomes. *Psychiatric Rehabilitation Journal, 29*(2), 173–180.

Powell, T. J., Yeaton, W., Hill, E. M., & Silk, K. R. (2001). Predictors of psychosocial outcomes for patients with mood disorders: The effects of self-help group participation. *Psychiatric Rehabilitation Journal, 25*(1), 3–11.

Rocchio, C. (1998). *The unvarnished truth, there is no cure for brain injury: Family news and views.* Alexandria, VA: Brain Injury Association.

Rolland, J. (1994). *Family illness and disability: An integrative model.* 1994. New York: Basic Books.

Rosenthal, M. (1987). Traumatic brain injury: Neurobehavioral consequences. In B. Chaplain (Ed.), *Rehabilitation psychology desk reference.* Rockville, MD: Aspen.

Santelli, B., Turnbull, A., & Higgins, C. (1999). Parent to parent support and health care. *Pediatric Nursing, 23*(3), 303–306.

Tang, M. (2001). Clinical outcome and client satisfaction of an anger management group program. *Canadian Journal of Occupational Therapy, 68*(4), 228–236.

Tomasulo, D. J. (2002). Stopping the "caregiver fatigue syndrome" through a self-support group program. *Mental Health Aspects of Developmental Disabilities, 5*(1), 16–21.

Wamboldt, M., & Levin, L. (1995). Utility of multifamily psychoeducational groups for medically ill children and adolescents. *Family Systems Medicine, 13*(2), 50–62.

Wiseman-Hanks, C., Steward, M. L., Wasserman, R., & Schuller, R. (1988). Peer group training of pragmatic skills in adolescents with acquired brain injury. *Journal of Head Trauma Rehabilitation, 13*(6), 23–38.

Zeigler, E. A. (1989). The importance of mutual support for spouses of brain injury. *Cognitive. Rehabilitation*, May-June, 34–37.

8

Interacting With Health Professionals: Family Needs and Perspectives

As families begin their journey living with a family member with a newly diagnosed chronic illness or severe disability, they will confront the impending reality of many necessary changes, difficult challenges, and continued demands. One of these demands is to develop a productive, collaborative relationship with health care professionals. Many family members may already have enjoyed a good relationship with a family doctor, but chronic illness and disability introduces the family to an entire new set of circumstances and the complexity of the health care team. Many new health care professionals, each with his/her own specialty, become involved in the treatment and rehabilitation process. Establishing a working partnership with these professionals is important if both the family member who is ill or disabled, and the family itself, are to achieve management and life adjustment goals.

The nature of the relationship between health care professionals and individual family members has changed considerably since the 1980s. These past years have witnessed massive changes in health service delivery systems (Krupat, 1986; Cooley, 2003). These changes in the professional-family relationship are attributed to two causes: the progress of scientific medicine and the focus on family-centered care as a framework for the delivery of health care (Harteker, 2003; Johnson, 2000; Wildes, 2001).

Older professional-patient models emphasized a fiduciary relationship, characterized by paternalism, complete control, an attitude of "I know what's best for you," almost total dependency, and one in which the professional is an advocate for the good of the patient (Nathanson, 1979; Wildes, 2001). These models were effective and expressed the truth that the physician's role, for example, was to act in the person's best interest. Unfortunately, the older models do not allow much room for individual responsibility in how people handle their own health choices. Paternalism is a recurring theme in the older form of the professional-family relationship, and this view tends to remove decision-making from the person and place it in the hands of the professional.

In the past, many health care professionals, moreover, perceived themselves almost as "pure" scientists, concerned only with the "facts," and therefore free from considerations of values in their interactions with consumers. Unfortunately, the traditional relationship models of professional-patient interaction focused solely on the medical component. The psychological impact of the illness or disability was not addressed, nor were other, important life adjustment issues of those who were coping with the experience (Roberts, Kiselica, & Fredrickson, 2002).

But the technological interventions of modern medicine, the emerging role of economics in medicine, and other scientific advances have all transformed the traditional professional-patient relationship (Wildes, 2001). A newer relationship model has been developed, such as the "market model," in which the patient is seen as an informed consumer (Wildes, 2001). Since a bureaucratic culture now plays an essential part in the delivery of health care, Wildes asks, "Are individuals true consumers in the current health insurance system?" (p. 9).

The progress of scientific medicine has affected the professional-family relationship to such a degree that individual responsibility and choice are valued. New treatment opportunities have emerged, demanding an understanding of both of the options: freedom of choice and the consequences of selection. The health professional is recognizing that the person must maintain freedom of control over his/her own life and destiny when significant choices are to be made. This relationship provides assurance to both the patient and the professional that each will retain his/her own integrity. The term *collaboration* assumes a new significance, since it is "not the process of conversion, but the development of new meanings by and for all parties involved" (Schilling & Stoller, 1995, p. 17).

Johnson (2000) reports that a combination of changing demographics, federal legislation, i.e., the Education for All Handicapped Children Act, the Mental Health Amendments of 1990, and the Individuals with Disabilities Education Act of 1990, increasing concern about rising health care costs, and the advent of managed care all suggested that relationship-based care with families improved individual family member health outcomes. A grassroots, consumer-driven movement also played a large role in shifting more attention to family-centered care. Literature about the importance of family involvement in health care appeared in the early 1990s, and highlighted collaboration with consumers as an essential strategy for creating change. Scholarly articles and emerging, hospital-based policies stressed that productive and responsible collaboration with family members in program development is key to implementing a family-centered system of care (Johnson, 2000).

The gradual shift from an "I'm in charge" approach (Lucyshn, Blumberg, & Kayser, 2000), to a more individual-centered style in which family members are questioned in an open-ended manner so that they can determine what is important to relate; the comprehensive attention in health-care to the role of the family to helping control costs and to affecting a more optimal change for the individual with a chronic illness or disability are realities that have provided an impetus to explore the health professional-family member relationship and to identify how their different roles can coalesce to form an effective partnership. This collaboration may facilitate both the adjustment of the family to the life and living responsibilities related to illness and/or disability, and can provide guidelines as to how the family can assist the individual family member who is ill or disabled to work on adaptive goals. While some of this information was discussed in Chapter 6, this chapter will focus on how the professional-family member relationship can be initiated, nourished, and enhanced, and how intervention strategies can be strengthened through productive collaboration. Also, to be discussed in this chapter as a foundation for what families and professionals need to do to develop their relationship, is an identification of family and professional relationship needs, and the problems and barriers to such a satisfactory relationship.

BARRIERS

There are several obstacles that may prevent a collaborative relationship between family members and professionals. From the initial diagnosis and throughout the entire course of treatment and rehabilitation, these barriers can occur and should be identified and managed if the family is to achieve an appropriate adaptation to the illness or disability experience. These obstacles are:

1. *The emotional reaction of family members to the impact of the illness or disability.* The suddenness of a disability condition, an unexpected diagnosis, or an exacerbation of illness symptoms can each cause a myriad of reactive and intense feelings within the family. Confusion, anger, and shock may be overwhelming emotions that create a continued state of fear and anxiety. These emotions are particularly evident

at the beginning of treatment when family members are thrust into an unfamiliar situation and are barraged with urgent decision making and often overwhelming information by feedback from the health care team. As they are experiencing these demands there is the accompanying realization that they are entering a new world that is, as expected, unknown to them.

All of these reactions as well as the sense of "strangeness" that is part of confronting the medical institutional structure, create difficulties when communication opportunities become available between the health professional and individual family members. Anxiety, for example, can inhibit the comprehension of important illness/disability-related information. Anger over either a perceived loss of control or loss of personal independence in decision-making becomes a resistant factor to the understanding of information. Family members may feel awkward to ask questions because of their unfamiliarity with the institution and treatment process. Of course, these reactive emotions are normal at the beginning of medical involvement with a chronic illness or severe disability. For any communication to be effective, the family will need time to sort through their feelings and begin to understand what has happened and what will occur. Also, family members may have a tremendous need to vent their anger, grief, fear, and powerlessness before they become willing listeners to important medical information.

2.   *Expectations of family members.* Because of the development of scientific medicine that has led to advances in diagnosis and treatment, people now expect medicine to cure people, especially their family members and themselves. Instead of medicine only ameliorating problems related to illness and disability, there is the expectation that the "miracles" that have become commonplace (Wildes, 2001) will also extend to a specific chronic illness or severe disability experienced by a family member. Family members may invest the health professional with magical powers. They may harbor unfounded hope. In his book, *False Hopes: Overcoming the Obstacles to a Sustainable, Affordable Medicine,* Callahan (1999) addresses this expectation when he states "Every dream must end even—perhaps especially—that of modern medicine . . . It has been fueled by the seemingly reasonable conviction that if we take up arms against a hostile nature, our ancient enemies—sickness, disability, and disease—can be overcome" (p. 25). Such expectations may also prejudice the complete acceptance of what is and what cannot be. Regardless of the caring posture and clear communication from the health provider, more improvement may be expected. The anticipation of the "cure" only delays complete attention to current management needs and prevents wholehearted endorsement of what the health care

team is attempting to do for the patient and family.

In addition to the obstacles, there are other family difficulties that hinder effective communication. Many family members, for example, may perceive themselves as terribly inadequate when confronted with the health care system. Communication is often not initiated, and even when initiated, it is often awkward and inadequate. Also, many families have "unfinished business" that has lingered in family life because of serious losses, disappointments, and the inability to resolve them or put them in context. An unexpected diagnosis or the sudden impact of a severe disability may revive issues of blame, guilt, and anger, which in turn stifles and impedes any opportunity to create a productive dialogue. Cultural considerations may also influence the interaction between health care professionals and family members. Certain ethnic groups may follow longstanding family traditions that frame how professional communication is enacted or utilized.

3. *Professional attitudes.* Specific circumstances that caused the onset of a chronic illness or disability may stimulate feelings of blame among providers towards family members. Because of issues of neglect and blame, family members may not only direct their anger towards another member, but also the health professional may also harbor such feelings towards the family. This may be especially true with families of children who have a chronic illness. When the disease becomes unexpectedly worse, and new symptoms appear, the professional may see the family as a cause of the problem, perhaps even as a barrier to the expected stabilization of the medical condition (Marshall, Seligman, & Prezant, 1999). Families of children who are mentally ill particularly may be objects of such perceptions. But these negative attitudes can create a distance between the family and the professional, and the provider may find it increasingly difficult to listen openly to family concerns and needs.

Professionals may also feel helpless when confronting an extremely difficult medical challenge with family members. In spite of medical advances, the downward course of an illness or disability may not be able to be stabilized or reversed. These feelings may be quite warranted, but may create a form of anxiety with the provider that inhibits frank and open discussion with family members. Though still pledged or committed to treat the medical condition in the best way possible, there may be an underlying sense of hopelessness that deters a more caring attitude towards the family. Family members of the elderly, for example, are often faced with the statement "What do you expect when they are old?"

4. *Professional communication.* The training of health professionals imparts a special language and its appropriate use communicates respect. But to those who are not familiar with this language, it can create high anxiety and a sense of helplessness among the uncomprehending (Hatfield, 1986). Language can also be used to control individuals, and technical language acts as a badge: it generates authority and sets the rules for response (Hatfield, 1986). Unfortunately, the continued use of professional jargon establishes boundaries that can be counterproductive. Family members may find it most difficult to understand what is being communicated and may feel that the language is a vehicle for control. These feelings, and the expected lack of language understanding, only exacerbates the distance between the professional and family. Semantic barriers can thwart productive relationships.

Marshall, Seligman, and Prezant (1999) have identified many other concerns that can impede the professional-family relationship, such as the discomfort professionals may feel in treating certain disabilities, the psychological and physical fatigue encountered in stressful occupations, and a preoccupation of the professional with personal concerns that tend to distract from careful listening. In addition, the reality of different world views derived from life experiences, and the consequent expectations that professionals and family member may harbor, can cause different perspectives on how health care should be delivered. All of these factors may place the health care professional in a poor position to interact comfortable and productively with family members.

FAMILY NEEDS

Pivotal to building a productive relationship between the family and health care professional is the latter's understanding of family needs, and the family member's ability to communicate these needs at specific times during the treatment and rehabilitation process. Previous chapters in this book have identified several types of family needs. Many of these needs are re-emphasized in this chapter, as they represent building blocks to construct an effective professional-family relationship. Several studies have reported family needs (Pieper, 1988; Wolman, Gorwick, Kohrman, & Blum, 2001; Hatfield, 1986; Gartner, 1988; Baxter, 1989; Scharar, 2002; Knox, Parmenter, Atkinson, & Yazbeck, 2000). Most of these studies focused on parents of children with disabilities or with family members who are mentally ill. Many of the research reports, however, identified common needs among families who are experiencing chronic illness or severe disability. Those needs stated as very important were:

- Have questions answered honestly, sensitively, and clearly
- Receive complete information on the family member's medical problems, treatment options, and medications
- Identify sufficient resources for the family member who is ill or disabled
- Assurance that the best possible medical care is being provided
- Assistance in managing health-related situations
- Help in organizing social support, when needed
- A willing listener to hear expectations about psychosocial well-being, acquiring independent living skills, education, and behavioral management
- Encouragement
- Increase confidence in problem-solving
- Suggestions for coping with a family member's behavior
- Information on how to obtain relief from financial distress
- Information on how to find respite care, when needed
- Information on how to contact people who are going through, as a family, a similar experience
- Interactions with health care professionals who:
  - listen attentively and with sensitivity to feelings of the family
  - respect the family's expertise and perspective
  - are sympathetic to family suffering
  - provide realistic hope and reassurance
  - encourage the family to set goals
  - apprise the family of what is going on
  - demonstrate to the family that they care
  - regard the family as an ally in the treatment of the family member
  - help family members to feel normal and comfortable when interacting with professionals
  - show an interest in what family members have to say and in how parents are managing
  - have pertinent information readily available
  - sharing of decision-making with service providers

The identification of family needs has been the foundation for the development of both assessment and intervention approaches described earlier in this book, and therefore a timely response to those needs by the health care professional can establish the groundwork for a productive relationship between the provider and family members. Thematic to all the family needs which have emerged from the many studies are core concepts stated by Harteker (2003) that pinpoint what is needed for an effective alliance:

- respect
- support
- strengths
- flexibility
- choice
- empowerment
- information

Importantly, if there is going to be an adequate response to what the family has requested when they are dealing with a chronic illness or disability, attention has to be directed to the specialty areas and accompanying distinct job responsibilities of health care providers. For example, alleviating financial distress, identifying sufficient resources, providing assistance in problem-solving, and contacting persons and families who are going through a similar experience in order to give insightful feedback are usually included in the duties of a medical social worker. Each provider, moreover, may provide different forms of support. An allied health professional, i.e., physical, occupational, or speech therapist, may give reassurance and praise during the treatment process; a physician may share needed, unbiased information that might allay some family anxieties; and a rehabilitation counselor might become an advocate for the family member to employers. All of these providers, whatever their professional contributions, can assist individuals and families "build on their strengths by participating in experiences that enhance control and independence" (Harteker, 2003, p. 3).

PROFESSIONAL NEEDS AND EXPECTATIONS

A health care provider has many personality-related needs and beliefs, some of which may interfere with family relationship building. The desire for or expectation of complete control when assisting family members with health care management concerns, or a longstanding bias that reveals the assumption that patients and their families can never be the experts in their daily experiences of providing care are two examples. In certain instances when a family is overwhelmed by the medical event and feels inadequate to take a role in responsible care giving, these may be valid expectations or beliefs by health providers.

If the medical treatment process is going to be managed effectively at home, and if family members are to become mangers of their own care, then they should acquire appropriate information. The family must become knowledgeable about the chronic illness or disability and its related stressors. There also may be difficulties encountered during the ongoing performance of care-giving responsibilities, and they are expected to speak out about their concerns and seek timely feedback. Having a stake in the outcome of efforts mutually shared by family members and health providers necessitates a family commitment and a respect for the health provider's needs or expectations. These needs may further include willingness of the family to be flexible concerning the treatment plans since unexpected changes may occur during the course of a chronic illness or severe disability. Also, families should be supported when they perceive that they have received inadequate care that has resulted in the creation of more problems and difficulties. A misdiagnosis or poorly managed treatment, for example, can elicit intense emotions and family members need appropriate information and other supportive assistance.

To be noted is that health professionals are not emotionally immune to a family member's severe medical condition. For various reasons they may feel in some way the grief, disappointment, and profound loss experienced by the family. The effects of a severe disability may prove to be irreversible, especially when there is the accompanying realization that the best care and most sophisticated technology is being provided. This realization has an impact on health providers and they may need for families to be aware of their feelings in such circumstances. Those who are daily involved with chronically ill people learn how to protect themselves from emotional pain or anxiety triggered by a particular medical event. But such protection does not necessarily thwart the need for awareness and respect from family members.

FAMILY GUIDELINES TO FACILITATE EFFECTIVE PARTNERSHIPS

Though the "perfect patient" and the "perfect family" in all domains of life and living are usually nonexistent, there are specific suggestions that can facilitate a working partnership between family members and health professionals. These suggestions are framed by definite responsibilities that individuals must undertake if they are to receive satisfaction when interacting with health care providers. Cohn (1987) has provided information on just what family members can do to establish this relationship:

1. Visits to health providers should be carefully planned, with questions the family wants answered identified and organized.
2. When a family member does not understand the information imparted by the provider, they must speak up and ask for a simpler explanation. The health care professional will probably welcome your participation.
3. Treatment planning is not the time to keep secrets or withhold information that may create obstacles to planning implementation. Full disclosure can prevent future problems.
4. Follow the advice provided by the health provider, and report immediately any adverse effects of therapy, complications from tests, or worsening of symptoms.
5. Ask about useful reading related to the chronic illness or severe disability.
6. The positive and negative issues that occur between the health provider and family members need to be discussed, not avoided. It is very difficult to communicate that a family member or the patient is unhappy with the way they are being treated. But communicating honestly, openly, and directly with the health professional may alleviate personal differences. The health provider should be viewed not as god-like, but as someone with special skills. This perception may help communication flow more naturally and feel less intimidating.

Trust between the family and health professional does not occur automatically, especially if the family has had prior negative experiences with health care providers or during the current times when the family wishes an active role in their member's treatment plan. Open communication is a beginning step towards building this trust, and trust is the foundation for effective collaboration.

HEALTH PROVIDER GUIDELINES TO FACILITATE EFFECTIVE PARTNERSHIPS

Because of the progress of medical technology, illnesses that were once fatal are now viewed as chronic. Consequently, there is an increasing need to be aware of the person's total life situation, including attention to the emotional, social, spiritual, and lifestyle adjustment issues of those who are directly experiencing the chronic illness and their family members (Roberts, Kiselica, & Fredrickson. 2002). Such a perspective extends the caring concerns of health professionals and introduces the importance of health care providers being aware of their own limitations, emotional and professional, to deal with these issues. The emotional issues that can play a decisive factor in the family member's own adjustment may be particularly challenging for the health care professional.

During the difficult periods of the course of a chronic illness or severe disability, moreover, some family members may become extremely distraught and despondent. The health care professional may feel defenseless, uncomfortable, helpless, frustrated, anxious, fearful, and emotionally distressed. To experience anxiety and discomfort is normal, but for the health care provider these feelings can become so intense and disabling that they hinder the helping process. In assisting many families in the treatment process who are experiencing profound feelings of loss and isolation, there is always going to be some agony. But if health care professionals have insights into their own defenses against grief and emotional pain, many feelings of discomfort can be better managed and controlled.

The ability to listen, respond, provide support, impart information at the family's level of understanding, and be open to the family's expression of feelings creates an atmosphere that fosters communication and eventually a mutually satisfying collaboration. Such communication also begins with accepting the family's view of problems related to care management. Also, to help family members build a partnership requires specific knowledge of how they have handled their losses historically and currently, as well as the ability to apply this understanding when the family expresses disappointment over the medical intervention, or appears hesitant to assume a necessary role when following a treatment regimen or when their emotions are raging and unrelenting. To be noted is that the family's response to the wishes of the health care professional is energized by the culture of the family, which may not be familiar to specific providers, and even such culture-driven expectations may be seen as a liability rather than an asset.

When there is the firm belief that a family-focused approach to the management of a chronic illness or severe disability can facilitate the achievement of rehabilitation and treatment goals, then health care providers may find it useful to encourage empowerment among family members. Empowerment includes the ability to maintain self-control, to be assertive, to develop expanded choices, and to become self-determined, if possible, when engaging in management and adaptive responsibilities (Bolton & Brookings, 1996). A climate must be established for the expression of these behaviors. For the health care provider, developing this climate requires, if viable and appropriate:

1. A willingness to hand over some responsibility for at-home management of the chronic illness or severe disability
2. The early identification of family strengths, and support of these strengths during treatment planning and throughout the management and rehabilitation process
3. Listening to opposing opinions and attending carefully to the family's views regarding their role in the treatment and rehabilitation process

Family members who believe they are empowered with regard to the care of the person who is chronically ill/severely disabled can gain a perspective towards the medical situation that is an important change from the feelings of isolation, abandonment, and anger that often accompany the experience. Providing families with a realistic sense of empowerment can create differences in how they adapt to the challenging losses implied in the assault on their sense of identity and integrity, and how they cope with social isolation, deal with financial consequences, and normalizetheir lifestyle (Pollin, 1995).

CONCLUSION

There has been increasing attention in the literature on approaches that call for a shift from provider-based, or expert-driven, services to a collaborative approach with a formal focus on the family context (Becker-Cottril, McFarland, & Anderson, 2003). Treatment and rehabilitation plans can be consumer directed and based, rather than "system directed and based" (Becker-Cottril, McFarland, & Anderson, p. 114). For such an approach to develop eventually into a collaboration between the health care provider and family members, the former must be present and concerned, empathic, and transiently identify with the emotional, social, and lifestyle concerns of the family and individual who are experiencing the chronic illness or disability. There are no established scripts, however, for how to learn to work with family members so that a collaborative relationship is established. Although self-awareness has been identified as the key to a successful health provider-patient relationship (Krikorian & Paulanka, 1982), additional skills are necessary if an alliance is to be created that assumes the family as a supportive and compassionate member. Frequently, when it is discovered that a family has a complicated and intense history resulting from neglect, malpractice, or other negative health care-related experiences, this reality must be confronted by the health care team with insight, understanding, and a plan to restore a more productive partnership.

SABINE: DEALING WITH MULTIPLE DISABILITIES AND DEATHS

Grieving is a journey that usually brings the conviction that there is no such thing as "closure." In her account of the multiple losses that she and her husband experienced, a mother describes how the death of each of her children was processed. During this process she met different roadblocks as well as welcome supports. Several of these obstacles and resources emerged from helping professionals and other family members. This personal statement identifies not only the hurdles and opportunities, but also provides recommendations that could make another's difficult journey somewhat smoother.

As the mother of four children, I have been in the unusual position of giving them life and then having three of them die. Both my husband and I have had to face many personal tragedies in our life, such as other personal losses and living through the ravages of war. However, coping with three disabled children has been the most demanding challenge of our lives. Our first child, a very healthy nine-pound baby girl, was born three years after my husband and I were married. A second child, a boy, was born two years later, and was a relatively small child at six pounds and a few ounces compared with our girl. He had extra digits on his hands and feet and no sucking reflex. That is all the doctors were aware of at that time, and he died after six weeks. The diagnosis was that he died of liver malfunction. At that time we decided to have another child as soon as possible. Our third baby was born thirteen months later and had the same symptoms as the second child. He also had extra digits, cleft palate, microcephalus, pyloric stenosis, and no sucking reflex. Those were the apparent problems. He also weighed only six pounds. The baby stayed in the hospital for three weeks and then went to another hospital. There he was diagnosed with Smith-Opitz syndrome. This syndrome had been only recently recognized and it was not known yet that there had been one case in our family already. People believed it could happen only to males and the chances were 25% per pregnancy for a couple like us. Apparently my husband and I have the same gene pattern, which is known to happen in only 1 out of 100,000 pregnancies.

The baby was released to our custody after a month in the hospital and we did not need help. We fed the baby by gavage through the nose directly into the stomach, which was not easy but certainly could be learned. From there on the baby needed attention 24 hours a day . For example, every two hours there was a feeding of one and a half ounces of formula, and I took up the job for almost a year before I realized that I was close to a nervous breakdown. Not because of emotion toward or against the child, but primarily because of lack of rest coupled with the demands of the rest of the family. At that time my mother-in-law asked us if she could take over the duties and have the child transferred to her apartment in a large, European city. There he was well taken care of, but made very little progress, remained spastic to a very high degree, grew tall but did not gain weight, and became difficult for this elderly lady to handle. But the love she gave to her grandchild made her bear the inconvenience and hardship. Due to her care, our son lived six happy years. He was the oldest recorded child with such a syndrome.

After his death, we decided to take another chance, and we had a baby a year after his death. Again, the baby had the same syndrome but this time the child was a girl. She looked normal at birth except for the extra digits, not quite as pronounced a cleft palate, and maybe microcephalus. She looked very much like our first girl, who was normal, and at that time we made the decision, which was not easy but most probably best for all including the first child who was ten at the time, to place the baby in an institution. She went from a hospital to a state school for only a short stay since they tried to use her for research and we did not approve. From there we brought her to an excellent small nursing home for young children with multiple birth defects. At that time we made a point that she should have the best of care but no heroic efforts should be made to prolong her life, which obviously was done in the first year of life to our third child. She lived eleven months. The diagnosis was pneumonia by food particles in the lung that unfortunately can easily happen with children fed by gavage.

In looking back on our ordeal, I realize that we helped the doctors; nobody helped us. We helped them learn more about the syndrome by our wanting to help medicine discover why it occurred. The only thing I think that wasn't done quite right by the doctors was how they told us what was wrong with the third child. After having had one child already who died, I think the doctors should have been more sensitive in breaking the news to us. Within five minutes after birth the doctor unbundled the baby and told us this and that was wrong and the child would never be normal and it most probably would have been better if it hadn't been born, but that is how it is. In other words, live with it! That was the only time I lost my cool and it took about a week to recuperate and accept that this could happen to us, since both of us are very healthy people and we never thought we might have any problem in having healthy children. The doctors and hospitals were generally very uncooperative in providing us with the records of our children. Also, I think it was insensitive and unprofessional for personal opinions, such as "cute baby" and "peculiar looking," to be entered on records. Only strict medical information should be put down.

Another difficult area for us was that we were criticized not only by friends and neighbors, but also by relatives for making the decision to have more children after we had one abnormal child. We more or less ignored their comments. We thought we had to make up our minds and do what we thought was best for our marriage. Both my husband and I love children tremendously and were not willing to give up after having one or two abnormal children. One reason we tried for a third child hoping it would be healthy was that the other two had died and we felt we could start all over. Nothing would have been more rewarding as having a healthy baby. We proceeded to live a normal life and didn't blame each other for having just one healthy girl. It seemed that everything was combined in our firstborn. She is healthy, very bright, and pleasant. She combines what we could look for in four children. So we are grateful we have her.

What was most difficult was the realization that with all the recent advances in medicine, nothing could be done to alter our personal situation. We were most fortunate to have one healthy child, which has been a stabilizing factor in our lives. However, having lost three children places an increased burden on us, since we are very concerned about the health and safety of our surviving child. What would we do if something happened to her? How could we cope? The way we have resolved this is to recognize that, in spite of tremendous stresses and strains in the past, we have been able to survive and cope. Therefore, we attempt to live our lives as fully as possible rather than constantly worrying about what may go wrong.

When we think about what we have been through, we recognize that it would have been impossible to survive if we did not have the support and understanding of each other as well as of several friends and family members who were able and willing to help in times of need. The constant physical care of our third child and the emotional drain that accompanied it was too much for any one person to bear. As parents of the child, we initially felt that it was our total responsibility. However, we soon recognized that it was more responsible to accept help rather than be unrealistic. Having lived with this experience and getting to know many other parents of disabled children, we feel that there are many things that could be done to initially ease the burden and reality of the situation. Most important to us would be the sensitivity and awareness of the medical profession to the emotional impact of having and caring for a disabled child. While there have been many excellent physicians and nurses who have worked with us, too often the busy schedule and high level of activity in medical facilities does not provide the opportunity or sensitivity required in responding to and supporting parents in crisis.

Another area that was very difficult for us was attempting to find those persons and resources who could help us during our time of crisis. It was most difficult having to phone and visit many agencies that seemed to be caught up in policy, procedure, and red tape, rather than personally responding to our needs. Reflecting upon our life, it is clear the reason we were able to survive was because we had the ability to do so and we made the decision that we would not be destroyed by our problems.

However, we recognize that even though three of our children have died, we still live with the impact of that experience. This is where parents who have lost children need a great deal of support in resolving the many issues that will remain for many years, such as should they adopt or how can they learn to modify the feelings about what has happed so they can live as full a life as possible. Both my husband and I recognize that our losses have taken their toll. We support each other, cry together and alone, and attempt to look ahead. Most important, we try to appreciate what we have rather than be bitter about what we have lost.

DISCUSSION QUESTIONS

1. In coping with the losses and caring demands emerging from children born with a severe disability, how were the emotional resources allocated within Sabine's family?
2. How was family balance regained following the death of each child, or was it regained?
3. If you were a helping professional and confronted with a family who must face intense caring and treatment decisions soon after the birth of their child with a severe, life-threatening disability, what further information would you need, and how would you intend to interact with the family?
4. How can traditions and cultural expectations be an asset or a liability?
5. Would your mother-in-law take care of your child if he/she hada severe disability?

SET 8: RAIN OR SHINE

PERSPECTIVE

One-way to gain perspective on the family challenged by a disability is to explore how families in general, and certain families in particular, function when life is ideal or not so ideal. Often, when families are in a state of crisis they lose contact with their pretrauma reality and tend to believe that, prior to a disability, their life was more functional, fulfilling, and rewarding. Conversely, they often believe that if the trauma had not occurred, that their life would be more fulfilling, satisfying, and rewarding. It is a perspective that can also be entertained by health professionals when they begin to connect with family members who are experiencing life with a disability.

EXPLORATION

1. List five qualities that define your family.
2. If you have experienced a severe illness or disability, were these qualities altered or changed?
3. If you were asked what are the abilities needed by a family to negotiate the perils of the disability experience, what would they be?
4. Are the responses to a disability different or similar to the responses to other traumas and losses?
5. Should divorce be considered as a reasonable alternative for individuals married to someone with a severe psychiatric disorder?
6. Should divorce be considered as a reasonable alternative for individuals married to a person who has Alzheimer's disease, AIDS, or a spinal cord injury?
7. Is the stress experienced by a family living with a member who has a mental illness different from the stress related to physical illnesses or disabilities? If so, in what ways?
8. Identify and discuss other familial factors that can intensify the stress associated with disabilities.
9. Assuming that self-help and informational programs were available and accessible to families living with a disability, do you believe that all families would benefit from these resources?
10. Some families and consumers of treatment and rehabilitation services cope with the illness and or disability experience by wanting, needing, and pursuing all relevant information. Other families see information as distressing and overwhelming. Do you feel that information is always helpful? If so, why? If you think it is not helpful, address the reasons.
11. If you were or are a person with a disability, what are or would be the sick-role expectations your family has/would have for you?

REFERENCES

Baxter, C. (1989). Parent-perceived attitudes of professionals: Implications for service providers. *Disability, Handicap and Society,* (3), 259-269.

Becker-Cottril, B., McFarland, J., & Anderson, V. (2003). A model of positive behavioral support for individuals with autism and their families: The family focus process. *Focus on Autism and Other Developmental Disabilities, 18*(2), 113–123.

Bolton, B., & Brookings, J. (1996). Development of a multifaceted definition of empowerment. *Rehabilitation Counseling Bulletin, 39*(4), 256–264.

Callahan, D. (1999). *False hopes: Overcoming the obstacles to a sustainable, affordable medicine*. New Brunswick, NJ: Rutgers University Press.

Cohn, V. (1987). Dealing with a silent doctor. *The Washington Post*, June 16, p. 8.

Cooley, W.C. (2003). The medical home-improving primary care for children with special needs. *Advances in Family-Centered Care, 9*(1), 4–7.

Education for All Handicapped Children Act, (1975) U.S. Department of Education, U.S. Government Printing Office, Washington, D.C.

Gartner, A. (1988). Parents, no longer excluded, just ignored: Some ways to do it nicely. *Exceptional Parent*, January-February, 40–41.

Harteker, L. (2003). Ensuring quality in cancer care through collaboration with patients and families. *Advances in Family-Centered Care, 9*(1), 8–13.

Hatfield, A.B. (1986). Semantic barriers to family and professional collaboration. *Schizophrenic Bulletin, 12*(3), 128–133.

Individuals with Disabilities Education Act of 1990. U.S. Department of Education, Washington, D.C. U.S. Government Printing Office.

Johnson, B. (2000). Family-centered care: Four decades of progress. *Families, Systems, and Health, 18*(2), 137–156.

Knox, M., Parmenter, T. R., Atkinson, N., & Yazbeck, M. (2000). Family control: The views of families who have a child with an intellectual disability. *Journal of Applied Research in Intellectual Disabilities, 13*, 17–28.

Krikorian, D. A., & Paulanka, B. J. (1982). Self-awareness: The key to a successful nurse-patient relationship. *Journal of Psychosocial Nursing and Mental Health Services, 20*(6), 19–21.

Krupat, E. (1986). A delicate imbalance. *Psychology Today*, November, 22–26.

Lucyshn, E., Blumberg, R., & Kayser, E. (2000). Improving the quality of support to families of children with severe behavior problems in the first decade of the new millennium. *Journal of Positive Behavior Intervention, 2*, 113–115.

Marshall, L. E., Seligman, M., & Prezant, F. (1999). *Disability and the family life cycle*. New York: Basic Books.

Nathanson, R. (1979). Counseling persons with disabilities: Are the feelings, thoughts, and behaviors of helping professionals helpful? *The Personnel and Guidance Journal*, December, 233–237.

Pieper, B. (1988). *In-home family supports: What families of youngsters with traumatic brain injury really need*. Albany, NY: New York State Head Injury Association.

Pollin, I. (1995). *Medical crisis counseling: Short-term therapy for long-term illness*. New York: Norton.

Roberts, S. A., Kiselica, M. S., & Fredrickson, S. A. (2002). Quality of life of persons with medical illnesses: Counseling's holistic contribution. *Journal of Counseling and Development, 80*, 422–431.

Scharar, K. (2002). What parents of mentally ill children need and want from mental health professionals. *Issues in Mental Health Nursing, 23*, 617–640.

Schilling, R. J., & Stoller, D. L. (1995). Opening the door to collaboration with physicians. In S. McDaniel (Ed.), *Counseling families with chronic illness*. Alexandria, VA: American Counseling Association.

Wildes, K. W. (2001). Patient no more. *America, 185*(2), 8–10.

Wolman, C., Gorwick, A., Kohrman, C., & Blum, R. (2001). Parents' wishes and expectations for children with chronic conditions. *Journal of Developmental and Physical Disabilities, 13*(3), 261–277.

Part III

Selected Family Issues

Emerging from the chapters in this book are four dominant themes that provide a further context for assisting families to adapt to the continued demands of living with chronic disease or severe disability. These themes are: *transition, loss, vulnerability,* and *affirmation.* With the diagnosis of a severe illness or disability family members experience a life and living transition. Accustomed patterns of family life are challenged; coping strategies must be developed to maintain an appropriate quality of life. Also, loss is a recurrent reality caused by many necessary changes in family life as well as the physical, emotional, and mental changes in the family member who is undergoing treatment and rehabilitation.

All families, moreover, are vulnerable to the unexpected or to the effects caused, for example, by addictive behaviors or mental illness. The illness or disability experienced by one family member can stimulate awareness in other members that there may be limits to one's capacities to manage adjustment tasks. But as a beacon casting a light on all of these issues flowing from transition, loss, and being vulnerable, is an affirmation perspective. This viewpoint generates an understanding that while illness and disability can cause despair, anguished concern, and rage, it can also open undiscovered doors to renewed opportunity, resilience, and encouraging hope. All of the book's chapters highlight the belief that families usually can find the strength to cope and continue with the business of living. Though changed in many personal ways, family members do not necessarily have to become victims. Interventions discussed in this book are directed to identifying these opportunities, to contain the impact of non-normative losses and to facilitate the process of normative adaptation.

Three of the chapters in this section focus on these four themes. Chapter 9 provides a framework for understanding family vulnerabilities caused by alcohol and related disorders. Chapter 10 presents the transition issues accompanying care giving and respite care. The personal statement by a daughter brings out the demands she and her mother faced when engaged in managing the difficult tasks related to care giving consequent to ALS. It is a poignant account that reveals the personal strengths and available resources that can be tapped during the most challenging of situations. Chapter 11 discusses the grieving process usually accompanying severe losses. It brings together existing literature, summarizes major approaches to understanding loss and grief, and offers a helping approach that both presents a beginning for the resolution of family loss and emphasizes the future life to live not limited by what was lost. The personal statement underlines this conviction and gives insights into how family members can maintain quality of life while experiencing the gradual loss of a loved one.

The final chapter represents the authors' reflections and considerations on family members who are everyday witnesses to the consequences of chronic illness or severe disability. It is an invitation to the health care team to be sensitive to and aware of the needs of the person and the family living with ongoing change and potential gains. Important for the reader, this chapter identifies several myths that may inhibit the treatment and rehabilitation process. Both the myths and the call for an identification of family expectations are intended to enhance the knowledge of those helping professionals who have contact with families while they undertake their job responsibilities. These professionals are actually partners with family members as they all embark on and continue this life and living journey of managing illness and disability. It is a journey that can have many positive results, especially when both the professional and the family are collaborating in assisting each other, and when the member who is ill or disabled discovers a better quality of life because of their mutual efforts.

9

Alcohol: An Illness, Disability, and Family Perspective

OVERVIEW

Alcohol use and abuse will always guarantee that many people, as well as their families, friends, and strangers, will become ill, disabled, and die. Ironically, the most serious and profound consequences are masked or distorted by the anticipated, as well as promised, joy and relief that has become the expectation of most people who use and/or abuse alcohol. Unfortunately, alcohol is marketed as a panacea to life's sorrow's and woes, but in reality it can be the cause of incalculable heartache, grief, sadness, and disappointment. In effect, alcohol is a major force in the assault on mankind, and the grim reality is that it often intensifies the vulnerability of many individuals and families. This reality is never reflected in advertisements that often promote alcohol as a solution to life's problems rather than a cause of them. In effect, alcohol is a "Trojan horse" and its abuse, or even use, is often a one-way ticket to illness or disability.

This chapter will explore alcohol use and it relation to illness and disability, while placing it in a treatment and rehabilitation context. Whether a person drinks or not, he or she is a potential direct or indirect victim of alcohol's toxic consequences. Serious concern about alcohol was expressed more than 116 years ago by Blair:

> The conflict between man and alcohol is as old as civilization, more destructive than any other form of warfare, and as fierce to-day [sic] as at any time since the beginning. It is not an exaggeration to say that no other evil known in human history has been of such vast proportions and lamentable consequences as that of alcoholic intemperance. As the whole past of the race has

---

*Some of the material in this chapter is updated and modified from Dell Orto & Power, 2000. Reprinted with permission.

been cursed by it, so its whole future is threatened with increasing calamity, unless there be a period put to its ravages. It is a peculiarity of this curse that it is developed by civilization, and then, like the parricide, it destroys the source of its own life.

But although alcohol is his special foe, it by no means confines its dagger and chalice to civilized man. Combining with the spirit of a mercenary commerce, this active essence of evil is hunting and extirpating the weaker races and indigenous populations of uncivilized countries from the face of the earth (Blair, 1888, p. ix).

When discussing alcohol, one must keep in mind that alcohol is a drug and its use and/or abuse can create personal and familial stress because illness anddisability are often direct and indirect consequences. As Fortstated more than thirty years ago:

Alcohol is our most widely used mind-altering drug. It is by far our hardest drug and constitutes our biggest drug problem in that it kills, disables, addicts, and makes psychotic more people than all the other drugs put together (Fort, 1973, pp. v–vi).

More recently Hutchins (2003) addressed some of the specific consequences related to alcohol and substance abuse: "Alcohol and illicit drug use are associated with many of this country's most serious problems, including violence, injury, and HIV infection" (p. 481).

These prior points generate a variety of perspectives, which are relevant to a discussion of alcohol and its relation to illness and disability.

PERSPECTIVES

The following perspectives capture the complexity and seriousness of some of the issues related to alcohol:

- There is a war going on that has more victims than most conflicts of recent memory. Just consider the death toll estimated at 26,000 per year. Every two years these numbers will approximate the loss of life of American military during the Vietnam War, and each year about eight times the lives lost in the World Trade Center tragedy. These numbers do not include the collateral damage of those injured physically or emotionally and the direct or indirect impact on their families.
- The ravages of alcohol-induced illness and disability are complex, long lasting, and often irreversible.

- The forces of alcohol's wrath and destruction are often driven by profit and commercial interests and often at the expense of the common good. Consider for a moment the advertising that is targeted to disadvantaged people living in economically depressed areas where alcohol is presented as a panacea to life's woes and a means to joy and happiness, while the consequences of its use and abuse are seen in the trauma centers and funeral homes.
- Although everyone is a potential victim, certain people are more vulnerable to the life-enhancing promises of alcohol-related advertising due to their pre-trauma or post-trauma cognitive, physical, and emotional conditions.
- Treatment and rehabilitation efforts and outcomes can be compromised by the presence of alcohol and other drugs.
- Alcohol may be used as a means of "normalization" and control when in fact it reduces control and increases the risk for additional problems. This is a critical point in those situations where a person may have limitations that are further compromised by the impairing consequences of alcohol use and or abuse. One disability or illness is not a guarantee that others may not occur.

SELECTED SITUATIONAL VARIABLES

When discussing the relationship between disability, illness, and alcohol, it is important to consider the many situational variables that can complicate the family's response to the situation as well as the implications for the treatment and rehabilitation process. For example:

- Was the injured person an alcoholic prior to the onset of illness or disability?
- Did alcohol have a role, directly or indirectly, in causing the situation?
- Was the family member in control or a victim (e.g., driver or passenger)?
- Was the person a nondrinker who was a victim of a drunk-driving situation? A crime of violence related to alcohol abuse?
- Prior to the trauma, was alcohol part of the family's lifestyle?
- Were there alcohol related problems?
- Did the person already have a disability, which was then complicated by a subsequent injury related to alcohol?
- Was alcohol use considered part of the normalization process?
- Is alcohol use a threat to the treatment and rehabilitation process?

The problem for many individuals and families challenged by alcohol is intensified when they realize that forces in our society have the power to impair, maim, and kill their children, friends, strangers, spouses, parents, and themselves. This may be the ultimate hangover. A direct result of this reality is the pervasive helplessness most people feel in controlling their destiny and the well-being of their loved ones especially when violence is a direct or indirect result of alcohol use or abuse.

VIOLENCE

Violence related to alcohol often results in very difficult and complicated emotional and physical situations (Harrison-Felix, et al., 1998). In a discussion of the relationship between alcohol and family violence, Shapiro (1982) indicated that family members are often the direct victims of violence resulting in trauma and disability. Kreutzer, Myers, Harris, and Zasler (1990) poignantly captured this theme of violence and the scope of the problem in an article poignantly entitled *Alcohol, Brain Injury, Manslaughter and Suicide.*

In addition to acts of physical abuse such as wife battering or shaken-baby syndrome, there are often other long-term and irreversible consequences, which may be a direct or indirect result of alcohol-induced violence by strangers or even family members. This can be a very complicated situation when a person is living with the stress of mental illness as well as violent behaviors. (Torrey, 1994). Unfortunately, when alcohol-abusing family members are the cause of a disability or loss, these situations often result in unforgettable realities that can be more consuming to the family than the forgiving, understanding, successful rehabilitation of the abusing family member who caused the injury or disability of a loved one, even if it was by default rather than intent. Unfortunately, alcohol use as means to improve a dire situation or enhance an enjoyable one can have many complications. This is especially so for people who are faced with multiple issues related to alcohol and disability.

ALCOHOL AND DISABILITY

While there has been an increased awareness of the problems related to alcohol use and abuse by persons living with illness and disability, alcohol might also be a major impediment in the treatment and rehabilitation process.

Consequently, individuals and families often find themselves experiencing the collateral damage related to the fallout from alcohol related injury and disability throughout the treatment and rehabilitation process. An added issue is how people, in difficult circumstances, attempt to regain control and restore what has been lost. When illness and disability are perceived as a loss of control over one's physical or emotional destiny, the stage is then set for some to cope with the concomitant stress, pain, grief, and depression by initiating or increasing their use of and dependency on alcohol or other drugs.

An irony of the substance abuse process is that even though it has resulted in a severe disability, some individuals may still rely on drugs and alcohol to cope with their physical and emotional losses (Greer, Roberts, & Jenkins, 1990). However, it is important to consider that among persons living with disabilities there are those who had a problem with substance abuse prior to the disability, as well as those persons who began using alcohol or other drugs following the onset of a disability. As one young man who is severely disabled said: "I do not drink to get drunk, I drink to feel normal again. When I drink I feel whole, when sober I am always aware that I am not. That is why my family does not say anything. They feel worse than I do and have told me they do not want to take away what little pleasure I have" (Dell Orto, 1990, personal communication). An additional point for consideration is how a family uses or abuses alcohol and how this directly or indirectly relates to the cause of illness or disability in the family. If a family's alcohol use is casual, there may be a negative reaction when the effects of alcohol abuse by a family member conflict with familial value systems and traditions. Frequently the family condones alcohol use because it is considered recreational, part of tradition, and less harmful than illegal drugs. This tolerant position can change dramatically if, under the influence of alcohol, a loved one is involved in a vehicular accident and becomes disabled or is the cause of an injury, disability, or death of others. It is within this transition from alcohol use to irreparable harm that most families find their ultimate agony, pain, and regret.

ALCOHOL AND BRAIN INJURY

One disability that reflects the many issues related to alcohol is brain injury. Faced with a reality that has been difficult to ignore, the field of brain injury rehabilitation, therefore, has given serious attention to alcohol (Corrigan, Bogner, & Lamb-Hart, 1999; Corrigan, 1995, 1996;

Corrigan, Lamb-Hart, & Rust, 1995; Delmonico, Hanley-Peterson, and Englander, 1998; Hibbard, Uysal, Kepler, Bogdany, & Silver, 1998).

The complexity of the problem and the synergistic relationship between alcohol and traumatic brain injury are summarized by Langley (1991) in a literature review related to the causal role of alcohol in the acquisition of traumatic brain injury (TBI), as well as its deleterious effect on rehabilitation. Langley concludes:

- Alcohol use is involved in the acquisition of 35 to 66% of all traumatic brain injuries.
- Alcohol is also a key factor in the failure of community reintegration efforts for many clients.
- Alcohol detrimentally affects functions associated with the prefrontal and temporal lobes including memory, planning, verbal fluency, complex motor control, and the modulation of emotionality.
- Alcohol use may further reduce the capacity for behavioral self-regulation for clients who have compromised prefrontal-temporal functioning due to traumatic brain injury.

An issue of *Brain Injury Rehabilitation Update* (1998) further focused on the consequences of alcohol use and rehabilitation:

> It is no secret that alcohol abuse and traumatic injuries often go together, and brain injury is no exception . . . those who do resume drinking may be compounding their problems rather than simply adding to them. The use of alcohol—even in a normal amount—is associated with poor neurological outcomes . . . (p. 1).

The implications of alcohol abuse are also clearly stated in the following statement:

> Alcohol abuse has been associated with TBI in approximately half of all occurrences. Whether the TBI is a direct result of alcohol or other substance use, or if it predates the substance abuse disability, the continued abuse of alcohol and other drugs can negate attempts at physical, social, and cognitive rehabilitation (SARDI, 1996).

In addition, Bogner and Lamb-Hart (1995) list the following eight points related to brain injury and alcohol and substance abuse:

1. People who use alcohol or other drugs after they have had brain injuries don't recover as much or as quickly as people who don't use alcohol or other drugs.

2.   Brain injuries cause problems in balance, walking, or talking that get worse when a person uses alcohol or other drugs.
3.   People who have had brain injuries often say or do things without thinking first, a problem that is made worse by using alcohol or other drugs.
4.   Brain injuries cause problems in thinking, like concentration or memory, and using alcohol and other drugs makes these worse.
5.   After a brain injury, alcohol and other drugs have a more powerful effect.
6.   People who have had brain injuries are more likely to have times when they feel low or depressed, and drinking alcohol and getting high on other drugs makes this worse.
7.   After a brain injury, drinking alcohol or using other drugs can cause a seizure.
8.   People who drink alcohol or use other drugs after brain injuries are more likely to have further brain injuries (p. 14).

These issues and their implications reflect some of the ongoing problems faced by people who are trying to get their lives together and are living with the many problems and issues related to and caused by alcohol. One such concern is dual diagnosis.

DUAL DIAGNOSIS

Another area of concern for health care providers as well as families is the coexistence of alcohol problems with other illnesses or disabilities resulting in dual diagnosis. In dual diagnosis situations, not only are families and individuals faced with the often complex and demanding consequences of illness and disability, but there are also added complications when alcohol abuse results in a unique set of problems and complications. (Basford, Rohe, Barnes, & DePompolo, 2002; Burke, Linden, Zhang, Maiste, & Shields, 2001; Doyle-Pita & Spaniol, 2003; Elliott, Kurylo, Chen, & Hicken, 2002; Ergh, Rapport, Coleman, & Hanks, 2002; Guthmann & Sandberg, 2002; Koch, Nelipovich, & Sneed, 2002; Temkin, Machamer, & Dikmen, 2001; Krause, Vines, Farley, Sniezek, & Coker, 2001; Kreutzer & Kolakowsky-Hayner, 2001; Scott & Popovich, 2001; Bombardier, 2000; Kilpatrick, Acierno, Saunders, Resnick, & Best, 2000; Livneh, 2000).

In effect, families are often faced with multiple problems when they have limited resources and options available to them. Regarding limited treatment resources and options, Sparadeo, Strauss, and Barth (1990) pointed out that, unfortunately, treatment opportunities for these dual diagnosis cases are very limited (p. 4).

This limitation may be due in part to the fact that many programs specialize in and focus on specific illnesses and disabilities, and do not consider or focus on alcohol, which may not be considered a priority or may fall outside of their scope of interest. However, the ongoing exploration of these issues is creating a better understanding of the problems, needs, and interventions (Moore & Ford 1996; Moore & Li, 1998; SARDI, 1996).

DUAL DIAGNOSIS AND MENTAL ILLNESS

In a discussion of dual diagnosis there are some unique concerns and issues related to mental illness, and the importance and complexity of dual diagnosis related to mental illness and substance abuse is stated in the literature (Doyle-Pita & Spaniol, 2003; Doyle-Pita, 1995; Drake, Mueser, Clark, & Wallach, 1996; Drake, Mercer-McFadden, Mueser, McHugo, & Bond, 1998; Minkoff & Ajilore, 1998; Mueser & Fox, 1998; Sharp & Getz, 1998).

Relating abuse to relapse Mueser (1996) stated:

> In addition, considering the strong relationship between both substance abuse and stress in contributing to relapse in psychiatric disorders, reducing these influences is an important goal of family intervention (p.28).

The challenging reality for families of persons who are mentally ill is that they are often overwhelmed by the demands and problems associated with the primary diagnosis of mental illness. Consequently, they may not be concerned about, aware of, or able to cope with the potential problems associated with the synergistic effects of mental illness and alcohol abuse, which could result in another physical disability such as spinal cord injury, brain injury, or both. In an opposite situation, a person with TBI is at risk for a secondary physical disability (Bogner & Lamb-Hart, 1995) or a psychiatric disability.

Hibbard, Uysal, Kepler, Bogdany, and Silver (1998) stated that TBI is a risk factor for psychiatric disabilities, and they expressed concern related to substance abuse disorders post TBI:

> Psychiatric disorders are frequent sequelae of traumatic brain injury. Long-term residual psychiatric sequelae pose challenges to community reentry and to quality of life and are often viewed as more seriously handicapping than the cognitive and physical sequelae of the injury itself (p. 24).

The potential for these sequelae is clarified when suicide attempts are related to mental illness complicated by substance abuse. It is important to realize that if a suicide attempt is not successful, there may still be irreversible physical and emotional consequences for the patient and the family.

An example of this is poignantly illustrated by the case of a young man who had a history of mental illness and alcohol abuse. He attempted suicide by jumping from a building. He survived with a severe brain injury complicated by a spinal cord injury. This was an overwhelming tragedy for the family who had successfully focused on and adjusted to the long-term demands of psychiatric disorder and a substance abuse problem; they were not prepared for the additional demands of TBI complicated by quadriplegia. A statement made by his parent can best capture this situation:

> One lesson we have learned is that we never again say it cannot get worse. It certainly can, but that also creates the possibility that things can also get better. In living with a physical disability as well as mental illness we certainly have experienced both and have a very different perspective. Now we are prepared for the worse, but expect and hope for the best and try to make it happen. If it does not, at least we were aware and not kidding ourselves (Dell Orto, 1990, personal communication).

While the drug or alcohol has had a major impact on the life of the individual and his family, it does not mean that the problem has been understood, managed, or eliminated. This point is illustrated by the fact that some people who have sustained a severe alcohol-related disability may still drink and/or drive. Consequently, they continue to place themselves and their families at additional risk for other problems and potential losses. The importance of this point is that there are stresses and residuals consequent to alcohol abuse that can be far more problematic than the alcohol abuse alone. The following case synopsis further illustrates this point:

> A person was referred for treatment with the presenting problem of adjusting to his brain injury. During the initial evaluation, a complex familial situation emerged. Prior to his injury, the individual was engaged in a problematic marital situation that involved alcohol abuse. After the divorce, the husband, while intoxicated, was severely injured as a result of an accident. He was hit by a truck and was comatose for three months. After a year of hospitalization and rehabilitation, he still had major cognitive difficulties and physical limitations. During this time his wife did not visit, wanted to get on with her life, and was on the verge of getting remarried. The complexity of the situation and financial considerations forced the couple to live together in a toxic

environment clouded by anger, bitterness, and resentment. Just as alcohol was part of the preinjury lifestyle, it became more of a problem during rehabilitation. This was manifested in physical and emotional abuse that culminated in legal action and charges of mutual assault and physical injury to the wife, resulting in a complex physical, emotional, and legal situation.

Another case synopsis, which illustrates the compounding nature of the effects of alcohol abuse, is as follows:

A middle-aged woman sought treatment for the presenting problem of chronic alcohol abuse and concern about her marriage. During treatment, her husband expressed his intentions to file for a divorce. When this occurred, the client, while under the influence of alcohol, went out for a drive and crashed into a bridge abutment. She sustained severe multiple traumas, was facially disfigured, and lost an arm and leg as well as sight in one eye. In addition, she needed many surgical procedures related to burns and her broken hips and legs. Her husband promised not to seek the divorce if she would sign all of their assets over to him. When this occurred, he left the country and disappeared in a remote part of the world where he had a supportive and approving family, leaving her destitute and suicidal. When asked about his actions he stated that he did not want to be married to a cripple—it was just not acceptable. This situation was intensified because the wife's motivation during a very painful and demanding rehabilitation process was to save the marriage. Her response was to drink heavily, placing her physical and emotional health in jeopardy and necessitating intensive alcohol treatment and rehabilitation.

Both these case summaries reflect the enormity and complexity of the disability experience for couples who are stressed by physical and emotional realities that are complicated and intensified by alcohol use. In both cases, the marital system was problematic prior to the onset of the injuries and collapsed when the added stress of the chronic disability experience took an additional toll. However, it must be pointed out that there are occasions when a problematic marital or familial system can be improved by initiating new behaviors and establishing more functional roles. This occurred in the following case:

A young couple had been married for five years and were on the verge of a divorce. This situation was a result of several years of individual alcohol abuse and domestic violence. The couple lived in the same house but led very separate lives. They had two children whom they both cared for. One evening the young woman was in an alcohol-related accident which was life threatening and was complicated by a severe disability. Her husband responded to the crisis by stopping his drinking, joining AA, organizing the family, and working toward the well-being and rehabilitation of his wife. A year later, they both were alcohol-free, intact as a family, and were appreciative of the gains that were a direct result of trauma and loss. The young man said it best when he stated, "I guess our lives were so out of control and distorted by alcohol that we both needed something serious to happen to get our attention." His wife said that know she feels better than she has in years and is very appreciative for the support efforts and actions of her husband which clearly demonstrated how much he cared.

CONCLUSION

The destructive power of alcohol use and abuse is very real. It may consume its victims and create a state of loss, failure, hopelessness, and helplessness. A person may die, be psychologically fragmented, be imprisoned by an illness or disability, and be the cause of a variety of personal and familial tragedies. In attempting to control these realities, families are faced with the task of self-examination, self-exploration, and often self-incrimination as they attempt to define their roles as part of the problem, or the solution.

For some families, their lives are complicated by the reality that they must be vigilant in their efforts to eliminate the disastrous consequences of alcohol while often being forced into roles and situations that are complicated at best. The challenge is not only to cope with an illness or disability, but also to live with the losses related to poor choices and often-irreversible consequences.

Contributing to this complex situation is the media, which has created norms slanted toward the hedonistic lifestyle made attainable by alcohol use and or abuse. On a daily basis, children, adolescents, and adults are bombarded by advertisements that create the image that alcohol is a vehicle to self-fulfillment, enjoyment, and excitement when, in reality, it is a potential shortcut to illness, disability, trauma, chaos, coma management, death, and familial collapse.

The challenge of working with persons and families living with a the demand of an illness or disability and the ongoing threats and consequences of alcohol abuse is mobilizing those resources and supports which can be stabilizing factors during an ongoing rehabilitation process.

To focus on the future benefits of treatment and rehabilitation without the development of viable alternatives to alcohol is ignoring the potential vulnerability of the population and the potential role of alcohol in a person's life. This is a significant issue because an individual who makes a commitment to treatment and rehabilitation often assumes that there is a chance to survive and attain a reasonable quality of life.

This is where organizations such as Alcoholics Anonymous (AA) have a great opportunity to address and meet the needs of persons and family living with alcohol related illness and disability.

If the skills cannot be utilized in the real world, relapse becomes a reality and those responsible for the design and expectations of the treatment and rehabilitation process must bear the burden of failure and not project blame completely onto their clients or the people they work with.

While there are many important issues related to the treatment and rehabilitation of persons living with illness and disability, there are also important issues related to the role of alcohol as a cause of illness, disability, loss, and death. How can we be content as a society that reacts to the problems consequent to alcohol use but ignores or minimizes the severity of the problems? Until we acknowledge and respond to the pervasive and causal role alcohol plays in the creation of illness and disability, we will remain victims of a double standard that decries the by-products of alcohol abuse but revels in the media distortion that presents people with a dream and delivers a nightmare.

JOHN: ATTITUDE IS EVERYTHING

The following personal statement discusses how, from the father's perspective, a family has negotiated the difficult journey that followed their son's injury caused by a drunk driver. It illustrates the implications of an injury to the dynamics of family life, especially how family plans may have to be delayed, and the importance of open marital communication if family adjustment is ever to be achieved.

Life sure deals some unexpected cards. I was convinced that I had gotten through the rough times in my life. After I married my second wife, life seemed almost perfect. She and her two boys and my son and I were becoming a happy family until the day that tragedy struck us. A woman who had been to a retirement party where she drank too much, got behind the wheel of a car, plowed into my son, and almost killed him. The doctors in the trauma center said he would live, but that we should start looking for nursing homes because his brain damage would cause him to be a vegetable. Why do they say things like that? I figure because they don't really know but they want to prepare you for the worst so you won't be shocked. When I think about it, I still get mad. It's a good thing that we didn't listen to them.

My first wife and I had my son when I was 21, so when he had his accident two years ago when he was 19, I was only 40, and my second wife was 35. Her boys were younger, of course, but we were definitely out of the babysitting stage. We were still young and free to do what we wanted without having to worry about the kids all the time.

After the accident, all that changed. We had a "child" who needed to be watched constantly at first. After a while, we tested him to see if we could leave him alone for longer periods of time. It wasn't a big problem because we're a family that has always done things together, so on the weekends we all worked on the house that we're now building on our property in Pennsylvania. During the week we had the most difficulty because both my wife and I work; she's a bank manager and I'm a mason. In the beginning, different people from our church would come and stay with my son. After a while, they needed to be there less and less. We're believers in the power of positive thinking. If you believe that someone can eventually be independent even when he's brain injured, you'll pass that optimistic attitude onto him. My wife was an independent child while growing up and she wouldn't let him act helpless. She kept expecting my son to take more and more responsibility. It was a little rough for her because at times she felt guilty about being hard on him, especially when the progress was slow. She went to talk to a counselor about it. The counselor helped her see that she couldn't fix him—that he would have to fix himself—that but it was okay to have expectations that eventually he would be more responsible. My wife's a backbone for this family. Sometimes I get very impatient if things move too slowly, but she convinces me that in time things will work out if we work at it. I know she's right. Even though my son's in a wheelchair most of the time, he can now stay alone, pick up around the house, and a couple of times a week he makes dinner. The good news is he's going back to school to learn about computers. Before the accident, he had no ambition to have a career. All he cared about was girls and sports. He definitely was not a great student. Now he still is not a great student, but he does have ambition. We know that it will be slow going. One thing about head-injured people is that even if they intend to do things, they can be very slow while doing them. One minute it seems he's forgotten what he said he was going to do. That's improving because he knows that he has to do his homework or he'll be embarrassed when he goes to class. It's good because he gets to be around other people and he needs that. If you were to ask him what's the hardest thing about life after the injury, he'd say not being able to walk, but if you ask me I'd say not having a normal social life. He wants a girlfriend in the worst way and was very depressed for a long time because he thought he'd never have one. Before the accident, he was a leader type, sure of himself, and he had lots of friends and girlfriends. Now, because he talks slowly and so softly he's very self-conscious, and for a long time he avoided people his own age. When he was in the rehabilitation center, he met girls who were head-injured also, but I know he really wants to meet a "normal" girl. As my wife says, "He was sweet before the accident and he's still that way and eventually he'll find someone who appreciates him."

I'm convinced the Lord works in strange ways. Since the accident, we're even closer as a family. The younger boys help their older brother. Of course, they fight like brothers, too, but they've learned compassion. We try hard not to neglect them because of their older brother's needs. We know that if we did, they'd resent him and we don't want that to happen. We haven't given up our dreams—just reorganized them. My wife was going to go to college full-time, and now she'll go part-time. We were going to build our house in 5 years, and now we'll take 10 years to build it. It's been interesting to design a house that could accommodate a person in a wheelchair. Even if my son leaves home and lives on his own, he'll always have a comfortable home to visit. If you want something and you're willing to work hard for it, you'll get it some way. Attitude is everything.

DISCUSSION QUESTIONS

1. How does surviving crises and making a new beginning create emotional vulnerability?
2. What is an adequate sentence for a person who kills someone in a drunk-driving accident? Who causes an accident that results in a brain injury?
3. Do you think that the suggestion made by the doctors in the trauma center that the father should start looking for a nursing home because his son would be a vegetable was helpful? Why or why not?
4. Discuss the impact of a brain injury when it occurs at various stages of childrearing.
5. How can the power of positive thinking be an asset, as well as a liability?
6. Discuss the positive and negative implications of the statement, "My wife was an independent child while growing up and she wouldn't let him act helpless."
7. .Give examples of how a person with a brain injury can perceive loss differently from parents or significant others.
8. What is meant by the statement, "We haven't given up our dreams—just reorganized them?"
9. Give examples of how the concept of working hard to attain a goal can provide hope as well as create frustration.
10. Should the makers and sellers of alcohol be liable for producing a dangerous product?

SET 9: ONE FOR THE ROAD

PERSPECTIVE

Since many injuries and disabilities result from vehicular accidents, it seems reasonable to focus on the cause of the problem as well as the effects. One consideration is that advertising often presents alcohol use as an integral part of daily life, which includes driving, recreation, socialization, and work.

EXPLORATION

In order to better understand the scope of the issue, do the following:

1. Go through a variety of magazines and select alcohol advertisements that you think create distorted images without attending to potential consequences.
2. Identify the groups of people you think would be most vulnerable.
3. Discuss the concept of responsibility in advertising.
4. Explore how potential consequences could be presented in the media, e.g., "This wheelchair's for you."
5. Should advertisers, brewers, and distillers be held responsible for medical costs associated with injury and disability consequent to drunk driving?
6. Should people with brain injuries be prevented from buying alcohol? Why or why not?
7. Which disabilities do you think could cause alcohol abuse?
8. How would you approach a person who said, "I lost so much as a result of my disability that I need to drink just to get by?"
9. If you or a family member were severely disabled, would you tend to use or abuse alcohol? What factors would influence your decision?
10. Should the media be limited in the kind of alcohol advertising they present to the public?
11. If you were a judge presiding over a case in which a drunk driver killed a 17-year-old and injured another 17-year-old who survived with a brain injury, what do you think would be an appropriate sentence? What would be adequate compensation for each family?
12. If a person under the influence of drugs or alcohol is injured while riding a motorcycle, who should be responsible for the medical costs? Should insurance be void?

REFERENCES

Basford, J. R., Rohe, D. E., Barnes, C. P., & DePompolo, R. W. (2002). Substance abuse attitudes and policies in U.S. rehabilitation training programs. *Archives of Physical Medicine and Rehabilitation*, 83(4), 517–522.

Blair, H. W. (1888). *The temperance movement or the conflict between man and alcohol.* Boston: William E. Smythe Company.

Bogner, J., & Lamb-Hart, G. (1995). Did I mention the teeth? *Brain Injury Association Journal, 3*(1), 12–15.Bombardier, C. H. (2000). Alcohol and traumatic disability. In R. G. Frank &T. R. Elliott (Eds.), Handbook of Rehabilitation Psychology. Washington, DC: American Psychological Association.

Editorial (1998). *Brain Injury Rehabilitation Update.* Department of Rehabilitation Medicine, University of Washington School of Medicine, Seattle, WA, Summer, 9(1).

Bombardier, C. H. (2000). Alcohol and traumatic disability. In R. G. Frank & T. R. Elliot, (Eds.). *Handbook of rehabilitation psychology,* Washington, D.C.: American Psychological Association, 399–416.

Burke, D. A., Linden, R. D., Zhang, Y. P., Maiste, A. C., & Shields, C. B. (2001). Incidence rates and populations at risk for spinal cord injury: A regional study. *Spinal Cord,* V39, N5, 274–278.

Corrigan, J. D. (1995). Substance abuse as a mediating factor in outcome from traumatic brain injury. *Archives of Physical Medicine and Rehabilitation, 76,* 302–309.

Corrigan, J. D., Lamb-Hart, G. L., & Rust, E. (1995). A program of interventions for substance abuse following traumatic brain injury, *Brain Injury, 9*(3), 221–236.

Corrigan, J. D. (1996). The incidence and impact of substance abuse following traumatic brain injury. In B. P. Uzzell, H. H. Stonnington, & J. Soronzo (Eds.), *Recovery after traumatic brain injury.* Hillsdale, NJ: Lawrence Erlbaum Associates, Inc.

Corrigan, J. D., Bogner, J. A., & Lamb-Hart, G. L. (1999). Substance abuse and brain injury. In M. Rosenthal, E. R. Grifith, J. D. Miller, & J. Kreutzer (Eds.), *Rehabilitation of theadult and the child with traumatic brain injury,* 3rd ed. Philadelphia: F.A. Davis.

Dell Orto, A. E., (1990). Personal communication.

Dell Orto, A.E. & Power, P.W. (2000). *Brain injury and the family: a life and living perspective,* 2nd ed. Boca Raton, Fl: CRC Press.

Delmonico, R., Hanley-Peterson, P., & Englander, J. (1998). Group psychotherapy for persons with traumatic brain injury: Management of frustration and substance abuse. *Journal of Head Trauma Rehabilitation, 13*(6), 10–22.

Doyle-Pita, D. (1995). *Addictions counseling.* New York: Crossroads Publishing.

Doyle-Pita, D., & Spaniol, L. (2002). *A comprehensive guide for integrated treatment of people with co-occurring disorders.* Boston, MA: Boston University Center for Psychiatric Rehabilitation, Sargent College.

Drake, R. E., Mueser, K. T., Clark, R. E., & Wallach, M. A.(1996). The course, treatment and outcome of substance abuse disorder in persons with severe mental illness. *American Journal of Orthopsychiatry, 66,* 42–51.

Drake, R. E., Mercer-McFadden, C., Mueser, K. T., McHugo, G. J., & Bond, G. R. (1998). Review of integrated mental health and substance abuse treatment for patients with dual disorders, *Schizophrenia Bulletin, 24*(4), 589–608.

Elliott, T. R., Kurylo, M., Chen, Y., & Hicken, B. (2002). Alcohol abuse history and adjustment following spinal cord injury. *Rehabilitation Psychology, 47*(3), 278–290.

Ergh, T. C., Rapport, L. J., Coleman, R. D., & Hanks, R. (2002). A predictor of caregiver and family functioning following traumatic brain injury: Social support moderates caregiver distress. *Journal of Head Trauma Rehabilitation, 17*(2), 155–174.

Fort, J. (1973). *Alcohol: Our biggest drug problem and our biggest industry.* New York: McGraw-Hill.

Greer, B., Roberts, R., & Jenkins, W. (1990). Substance abuse among clients with other primary disabilities: Curricular implications for rehabilitation education. *Rehabilitation Education, 4,* 33–44.

Guthmann, D., & Sandberg, K. (2002). A relapse prevention with deaf persons. *Journal American Deafness and Rehabilitation Association, 35*(1), 15–24.

Harrison-Felix, C., Zafonte, R., Mann, N., Dijkers, M., Englander, J., & Kreutzer, J. (1998). Brain injury as a result of violence: Preliminary findings from the traumatic brain injury model systems. *Archives of Physical Medicine and Rehabilitation, 79*(7), 730–737.

Hibbard, M., Uysal, S., Kepler, K., Bogdany, J., & Silver, J. (1998). Axis 1 psychopathology in individuals with traumatic brain injury. *Journal of Head Trauma Rehabilitation, 13*(4), 24–39.

Hutchins, E., (2003). Ensuring Substance Abuse Services for Families. In H. Wallace, G. Green, & K. Jaros (Eds.), *Health and welfare for families in the 21st century.* Sudbury, MA: Jones & Bartlett.

Kilpatrick, D. G., Acierno, R., Saunders, B., Resnick, H. S., & Best, C. L. (2000). Risk factors for adolescent substance abuse and dependence: Data from a national sample. *Journal of Consulting and Clinical Psychology, 68*(1), 19–30.

Koch, D. S., Nelipovich, M., & Sneed, Z. (2002). Alcohol and other drug abuse as coexisting disabilities: Considerations for counselors serving individuals who are blind or visually impaired. *RE:view, 33*(4), 151–159.

Krause, J. S., Vines, C. L., Farley, T. L., Sniezek, J., &Coker, J. (2001). An exploratory study of pressure ulcers after spinal cord injury: Relationship to protective behaviors and risk factors. *Archives of Physical Medicine and Rehabilitation, 82*(1), 107–113.

Kreutzer, J. S., & Kolakowsky-Hayner, S. A. (2001). Alcohol & drug use after spinal cord injury: Institution: VCU/MCV Spinal Cord Injured (SCI) Model System, Report Number: H133N50015, Virginia Commonwealth University, Department of Physical Medicine and Rehabilitation.

Kreutzer, J. S., Myers, S. L., Harris, J. A., & Zasler, W. D. (1990). Alcohol, brain injury, manslaughter and suicide. *Cognitive Rehabilitation, 8*(4), 14–18.

Langley, M. J. (1991). Preventing post injury alcohol-related problems: A behavioral approach. In: B. T. McMahon & L. R. Shaw (Eds.), *Work worth doing: Advances in brain injury rehabilitation.*Orlando, FL: Paul M. Deutsch Press.

Livneh, H. (2000). Psychosocial adaptation to spinal cord injury: The role of coping strategies. *Journal of Applied Rehabilitation Counseling, 31*(2), 3–10.

Minkoff, K., & Ajilore, C. (1998). *Co-occurring psychiatric and substance abuse disorders in managed care systems: Standards of care, practice guideline, workforce competencies, and training curricula.* Rockport, MD: Report Center for Mental Health Services Managed Care Initiative.

Moore, D., & Ford, J. (1996). Policy responses to substance abuse and disability: A concept paper. *Journal of Disability Policy Studies, 7*(1), 91–106.

Moore, D., & Li, L. (1998). Prevalence and risk factors of illicit drug use by people with disabilities. *The American Journal on Addictions, 7*(2), 93–102.

Mueser, K. (1996). Helping families manage severe mental illness. *Psychiatric Rehabilitation Skills, 1(2),, 21–42.*

Mueser, K., & Fox, L. (1998). Dual diagnosis: How families can help, *Journal of the California Alliance for the Mentally Ill,* 9, 53–55.

SARDI (1996). *Substance abuse, disability and vocational rehabilitation, research and training center on drugs and disability.*Dayton, OH: Wright State School of Medicine.

Scott, C. M., & Popovich, D. J. (2001). Undiagnosed alcoholism & prescription drug misuse among the elderly. *Caring, 20*(1), 20–23.

Sharp, M., & Getz, J.(1998). Self process in co-morbid mental illness and drug abuse. *American Journal of Orthopsychiatry, 68*(4), 639–644.

Shapiro, R. (1982). Clinical approaches to family violence. *The Family Therapy Collection.* Rockville, MD: Aspen Press.

Sparadeo, F. R., Strauss, D., & Barth, J. T. (1990). The incidence, impact and treatment of substance abuse on head trauma rehabilitation. *Journal. of Head Trauma Rehabilitation,* 5(3), 1–8.

Temkin, N. R., Machamer, J. E., Dikmen, S. S. (2001). Utility of a composite measure to detect problematic alcohol use in persons with traumatic brain injury. *Archives of Physical Medicine and Rehabilitation, 82*(6), 780–786.

Torrey, E. F. (1994). Violent behavior by individuals with serious mental illness. *Hospital and Community Psychiatry, 45,* 653–662.

10

Challenges and Issues in Caregiving and Respite Care

PERSPECTIVE

Caregiving and respite care are life transitions and vital forces for both the caregiver and care recipient who are engaged in negotiating the often-complex demands related to illness and/or disability experiences. These life transitions, many of which require caregiving as well as respite care, can occur any time during the life span (Brandstater & Shutter, 2002; Eaves, 2002; Dowling & Dolan 2001; Cocks, 2000; Breckbill & Carmen, 1999), and are more the rule rather than the exception during the aging process which creates its own unique caregiving needs and expectations (Hartke & King, 2002; Kriegsman, Penninx, & vanEijk, 1995; McGrath, Mueller, Brown, Teitelman, & Watts, 2000; Shannon, 2001).

An ongoing challenge during major life transitions is to attend to complex individual needs while shoring up collective resources and meeting the current and emerging needs of the family. This is not an easy task and often presents as many problems as solutions, especially for the caregivers who are often faced with expectations that far exceed their resources (Bakas & Burgener, 2002; D'Asaro, 1998; Smith & Smith, 2000; Sander, Sherer, Malec, High, Thompson, Moessner, & Josey (2003); Newsom & Schulz, 1998).

It is often easier to understand the philosophy and principles of caregiving and respite care than to apply and integrate them into many family settings and situations. This is often due to the complex emotional forces that can influence the process and the historical experiences that impact the ability of families to assume diverse and complicated

---

Some of the material in this chapter is based on, updated, and modified from 'Dell Orto & Power, 2000 and Power, Dell Orto, & Gibbons, 1988. Reprinted with permission.

caregiving roles. For some families there are traditions that create a common ground. They are clear on what is expected and have the skills and supports to negotiate the caregiving/respite care experience. For others, it is a very alien world and most unsettling experience. Often this is related to ongoing change related to caregiving.

Given the probability or eventuality of most families being in some form of a caregiving role during their lifetime, it is prudent, if not wise, for families to consider and actively prepare for this role in times of less stress and tranquility, rather than waiting to assess and test their skills and resources at a time of crisis.

This chapter will discuss principles and issues of caregiving and explain selected topics that contribute to the complexities of caregiving. These include gender, role flexibility, stress, wellness, marital relationship and abandonment. Added to these issues are explanations of extraordinary care, compensation, and respite care.

CAREGIVING

Traditionally, caregiving has been viewed as an expectation from those who are in traditional caregiving roles, e.g., women, parents, spouses, significant others, children, relatives, etc. More recently caregiving has been extended to those persons who provide such care on a compensated or volunteer basis. Such caregiving has become the focus of ongoing discussion and debate related to the need for increased caregiver support (Angell, 1999; Arno, Levine, & Memmott, 1999; Fredriksen & Scharlach, 1999; Levine, 1998, 1999; Ergh, Rapport, Coleman, & Hanks, 2002).

While there are some families who have reliable support systems, some families do not have these assets and must do the best with what they have. Sometimes this is not adequate to meet the demands of the situation. Also, in today's mobile and geographically dispersed society, families may have to rely on people who are not family members to provide caregiving support and resources.

PRINCIPLES AND ISSUES

Underlying the illness and disability experience are selected principles and issues that may influence how the family responds to caregiving and respite care, including:

- No family is ever completely prepared for the demands, implications, and changes relate to the caregiving process.
- Illness and disability changes a family and challenges its caregiving skills, values, supports, and resources.
- Caregiving brings out the best and worst in individuals and in families.
- Illness, disability, caregiving, and respite care demands can deplete family resources as well as create them.
- Often the only caregiving or respite care support available is the family, and it may not be helpful, welcome, or appreciated.
- Not everyone has a family that can be relied on for all situations and for all members.
- Not all families are capable of responding to the current and emerging caregiving and respite care needs of an ill, disabled, or aged family member.
- New caregiving skills and respite care options are needed by the family to meet the ongoing challenges created by the illness, disability, or aging of a member.
- Not everyone is going to improve, even under the best of circumstances or with the best of care.
- Sometimes the best treatment and rehabilitation programs do not meet family expectations.
- Coping with loss, change, illness, disability, and aging is an ongoing developmental process for the individual and the family.
- Caregiving and respite care often make the difference between coping and deterioration.
- Not all family members currently love or care for the person in need, even if they have in the past.
- Often families survive by creating hope based upon desperation and not reality.
- Some individuals are treated better by strangers than by family members.
- Existing health care resources can help and/or hinder adjustment.
- Financial resources can solve some problems and create others.
- Families may not reciprocate for the caregiving or respite care they have received from their family or significant others.
- Family history and traditions can be assets or liabilities.

These points are emphasized as selected examples of some of the issues, forces, and dynamics that families may have to face while attempting to understand and meet the caregiving needs of their family member. Common to many caregivers is the feeling that they have lost or marginalized their own lives and needs while losing many of the activities and people that once provided a sense of balance and support.

A frequent lament of many families living with illness or disability is that they are not adequately prepared for the demands related to the caregiving process and are in need of more support, especially in the respite care domain. This situation exists, in part, because some health care and rehabilitation systems are designed to provide treatment based on the assumption, presumption, and/or hope that at some point the individual, family, or significant other will develop the physical, financial, and emotional resources necessary to deal with the torrent of demands following an illness or disability experience. Often this is not the case, and families are left on their own and may feel abandoned or let down by the health care of their family system.

The following case illustrates many of the principles and issues of caregiving and shows how one family had as part of its tradition to take care of family members in sickness and in health, as well as provide palliative care.

The family consisted of a mother, a father, three sons, and a daughter. The parents immigrated to the United States in the 1920s. They pursued "the American dream" through total parental sacrifice and focused on the well-being of their children and on the desire that they become educated and productive members of society. However, their cultural background valued education for the sons, whereas the daughter's role was to stay home to take care of the family.

Eventually, the sons got married and started families and careers of their own. At this point, it was possible for the daughter to begin to develop a life of her own. She was academically talented and had a chance to go to college as well as an offer for marriage. While she wanted to get married, it required that she move 1500 miles away from her parents. However, the illness of her mother created a situation where she was expected to, and chose to, care for her mother because (1) she was a woman, (2) she was at home, (3) she was not married, and (4) this was the way it was traditionally done in their culture. More important, this was what she wanted to do and was happy about it. Therefore, her role emerged as caretaker for her ill mother, who suffered a stroke, and her father, who had Alzheimer's disease. Her mother began to deteriorate and needed continuous care, which tested the resiliency of the family and its ability to provide respite care to each other. Not only did all the sons share in the financial aspects of sustaining their sister and parents, but also their wives equally divided the tasks of caring for their elderly parents. They worked from the framework of a cultural tradition, used family conferences, designated the tasks, and identified who would be responsible for specific tasks. What was most impressive about this family is that even considering that they had the advantages of geographically centralized living arrangements, they had a functional attitude that was demonstrated in the willingness to do more than was expected or designated as their tasks. An example was how one daughter-in-law provided constant care for three weeks while another daughter-in-law cared for a sick child. She did not expect that the time should be made up and did not accept it when the offer was made.

This high level of functioning continued for seven years, at which time the mother died, and then for another 5 years until the father died. This created a situation where the daughter was left alone without a job or income. A family meeting was held and the decision was made to give the family home to the daughter and to provide her with a weekly income for the years she sacrificed for the family. Unfortunately, this was a short-lived pause, because the wife of one of the brothers became terminally ill and the daughter resumed her role as caregiver. When her sister-in-law died, her brother had a heart attack, moved in with her and stayed for two years until he died. At this point, the daughter became ill and was cared for by her sister-in-law until her death. At her funeral her brothers and sisters-in-law said: "We lost a wonderful person who taught us how to be the best people we can be under very difficult circumstances and showed us how to live and enjoy life. This is a most precious gift."

COMPLEXITIES OF CAREGIVING

For families with complex conditions there are many problems to be considered and addressed. Often these are related to the intensification of the responsibilities and consequences of caregiving. Caregiving has many dimensions, moreover, and some families find themselves concurrently facing problems in several domains. While any one of these problem areas may be manageable for some families, the cumulative effect of several or many at the same time can be very problematic and often overwhelming. Some of the problems encountered by caregivers were identified by Kahana, Biegel, and Wykle (1994), as follows:

1. Coping with increased needs of the dependent family member caused by physical and/or mental illnesses
2. Coping with disruptive behaviors, especially those associated with cognitive disorders or mental illness such as dementia or schizophrenia

3. Restrictions on social or leisure activities
4. Infringement on privacy
5. Disruption of household and work routines
6. Conflicting multiple role demands
7. Lack of support or assistance from other family members
8. Disruptions of family roles and relationships
9. Lack of sufficient assistance from human service agencies and agency professionals

Furthermore, on occasion families may be put in the position of having to choose between their emotional and physical stability and the care of an ill or disabled member. For example, some family members may want to keep the person at home, while others may want to place the person in a long-term care facility. In such cases, caregiving options can often make the difference between a family's ability to make lifetime care choices from a position of strength rather than default. The complexity of these choices is addressed by Jarman and Stone (1989):

> Some parents may find they simply cannot provide the care their loved one needs, no matter how hard they try. At this point they agonize over the right decision, and are forced to acknowledge that they cannot make it "all better" for their injured child. Considering placement and alternative living options becomes a very difficult decision-making process for these parents (p. 32).

This situation can be more complicated when caregivers are faced with multiple demands with limited options. An example of this is the situation where a family is caring for a parent with Alzheimer's disease. This situation worked very well for several years till the daughter-in-law was severely injured in a car accident. At that time the son tried to take care of both his wife and his mother, but could not do it and had to make the very difficult decision of placing his mother in a nursing home. This was most difficult because he wanted to take care of both his wife and his mother, but a bad back and a heart condition as well as the input from his doctor and other family members precluded this option.

Commenting on the complex demands of caregiving process Stober-Larsen (1998) stated:

> As the ill relative becomes more dependent, the caregiver's tasks become more complex and time-consuming and it is not uncommon for caregivers to feel they are devoting their entire lives to caregiving (p. 26).

Further, in addressing another complexity, the demands and costs of caregiving, Biegel (1995) stated:

> Research on the effects of caregiving shows very clearly that caregiving is not without costs to the caregiver. Many families report caregiving to be an emotional, physical, and at times, financial burden (p. 146).

Because there is the expectation that some families will continue to devote their resources and engage in the demands of caregiving when they have not been given the support they need to provide care, often under very harsh conditions, this is an important point. Also, Gillen, Tennen, Affleck, and Steinpreis (1998) stated that even if supports are in place during hospitalization or rehabilitation, they may not be the best fit for the caregiver. This may result in a situation where the family is forced to use what is available—good, neutral, or bad.

In some situations, while the effort at caregiving is being made it may not be worth the cost to all involved. Gillen, Tennen, Affleck, and Steinpreis (1998) commented that in addition to adverse outcomes such as suicide, hospitalization, and divorce, depression may be associated with impaired caregiving, or caregiving that is so overwhelming it is not in the best interest of the patient to be in such an environment.

GENDER ISSUES AND ROLE FLEXIBILITY RELATED TO CAREGIVING:

Traditionally, the woman has been designated by choice, tradition, or default to be the provider of "nurturance and care" (Zeigler, 1989). In effect, women often become the caregivers, even if they are not the best people for the job. Their efforts and energies may be better placed in other areas. Zeigler (1989) comments:

> Strong emotional attachment to loved ones and the nurturing demands placed on women by their family members may create significant stress. Although society assigns nurturing responsibilities to women in crisis situations, little value is place on these services. The care recipient receives the benefit, often to the detriment of the caregiver's physical and mental health (p. 54).

While there have been gains made in the emergence of new caregiving roles for both women and men, there is still concern regarding making the role modifications necessary to respond to the specific needs of a loved one or the complex demands of the respite care process (Yee & Schultz, 2000; Christensen, Stephens, & Townsend 1998). Therefore, role flexibility is key to the ability to alter personal goals, aspirations, and needs for the benefit of the total family system. While difficult in the best of circumstances, role flexibility is almost impossible when elements of personal and familial dysfunction foster role rigidity, interpersonal stress, and pervasive chaos.

Even successful caregiving can be a double-edged sword. Some caregivers are able to negotiate the demands of caregiving because they see it for a limited time with an end in sight. For others the process is complicated by their need to hold on and make things better, all the while feeling distressed because they want to let go and get on with their lives. Also of note is the dramatic change of roles that can be an additional stressor in the caregiving experience. These role shifts can occur when an affectionate, responsible spouse becomes a demanding, irresponsible patient, and the loving, caring spouse becomes a resentful caregiver who sees caregiving more as a curse than an opportunity. Often these situations create stress for all involved.

AREAS OF STRESS RELATED TO CARGIVING:

An overwhelming perception of burden, accurate or not, may create stress and frustration on the part of those caregivers who are in desperate need of services (Kosciulek & Lustig, 1998). Lustig (1999) has also independently discussed the role of stress and its impact on the family:

> Family stress is the result of an imbalance between the demands placed on the family and capabilities of the family to deal with the stressor. When the demand-capability imbalance is pronounced, the family may experience maladjustment. The ability of the family to successfully adjust to a stressor is determined by the family's vulnerability, resources, appraisal, problem solving and coping (p. 26).

The following examples provide some examples of issues and stressors related to caregiving, and the importance of respite care:

1. A grandfather living with a stroke who cannot regulate bodily functions is agitated and has to be constantly supervised because he has hit family members, including the children. Enormous stress is placed upon the wife, children, and grandchildren because he acts like a child and requires ongoing care that has resulted in ongoing family conflict and stress because some want to keep him at home since he was a great father and grandfather till the stroke. Other family members

want to have him placed in a care facility because it was too much work and effort and all of the care issues are getting in the way of their lives.

2.   The elderly parent who has a child with a severe developmental disability and was able to manage with the help of her daughter until the daughter was diagnosed with cancer and became another patient in the family rather than a caregiver.

3.   A woman who has Parkinson's and cannot get help from her husband due to his mental illness. This is complicated by the constant turnover of workers and lack of a supportive family. She stated that her family would rather complain than help.

What these examples have in common is the intensity of a complex situation, which has resulted in increased familial distress, and has created the potential for accelerated family needs, problem resolution, and support. Active interventions in such situations enable the family to develop a pause in the caregiving process, while assessing their needs and replenishing their resources. As a result, family members may be able to renegotiate their familial roles and establish new ones that are more conducive to coping, rejuvenation, and survival.

Schultz and Quittner (1998) commented on the commonality of stress for the care recipient and caregiver:

> The dominant conceptual model for caregiving assumes that the onset and progression of chronic illness and physical disability is stressful for both the patient and caregiver and, as such, can be studied within the framework of traditional stress-coping models. Indeed, some researchers have likened caregiving to being exposed to a severe, long-term chronic stressor(p. 107). Contributing to stress in caregiving are the issues of abandonment and the provision of extraordinary care.

ABANDONMENT

In addition to the ongoing stress related to caregiving, families may have to deal with actual or perceived abandonment by family, friends, and the health care system. One area that is of particular concern is the loss of family support in times of need. Gardner (2002) discussed the impact of the loss of support and how it relates to isolation:

> Since many individuals lose most or all of their friends over time, the loss of family support—especially that of the primary care and support giver—would be a major blow to his/her support network. It would isolate the individual further, leaving the person to fend for him/herself in a world that already poses significant challenges (p. 41).

In a time of health care crisis some family members may decide that their lifestyle or current demands are not compatible with the caregiving process. Others may be dealing with unfinished family business, and their lack of concern or action may be an indirect way of addressing these issues. These situations are made more painful when the person in current need has been a caregiver for others and must face painful disappointment at a time of desperate and often anticipated support and relief. This is further complicated when the systems that are supposed to help contribute to the problem rather than help solve it.

Commenting on the impact of abandonment by the health care system, Levine (1999) stated:

> I feel abandoned by a health care system that commits resources and rewards to rescuing the injured and ill but then consigns such patients and their families to the black hole of chronic custodial care (p. 1588).

Theoretically, the availability of caregiving options and respite care programs should reflect a match between need and resources. Unfortunately, the need most often is in excess of the resources.

EXTRAORDINARY CARE

Many families engaging in traditional caregiving may not be prepared for the unique demands related to extraordinary care. Focusing on caregiving in difficult situations, Biegel (1995) stated:

> Caregiving due to chronic illness and disability represents something that, in principle, is not very different from traditional tasks and activities rendered to family members. The difference in real terms, however, is that caregiving in this situation represents the increment of extraordinary care that goes beyond the bounds of usual care (p. 146).

Under the demands of extraordinary care, family members are often faced with the additional burden of stress. In these situations, caregivers may expect or hope that other family members will sense the stress and voluntarily demonstrate concern, both in word and in action. Unfortunately, if this does not occur, resentment and disappointment may result in family conflicts and cutoffs. To prevent or minimize this, it would be helpful if caregivers had the opportunity to learn how to express their needs and expectations rather than relying on the intuition or sporadic goodwill of others.

There is an added stressor for families when the family member's behavior becomes destructive, aggressive, or dangerous. In these situations, the person changed by illness or disability may be perceived as a stranger whose behavior makes an out-of-home placement attractive and home care problematic. Often families are so burdened and frustrated that they have "burnout," and make alternate living arrangements based on their frustration and desperation, or they are reluctant to seek help until they are at the point of physical, financial, and emotional exhaustion. At this point, there is often great need and efforts should be made to try to stabilize the patient and the family. One option is through a combination of outreach groups, as discussed in Chapter 7, and ongoing life support seminars which can provide a forum for skill development and ongoing peer support.

If families are not in a position to provide ordinary or even extraordinary care, someone will have to fill the void—often at inflated and unreasonable costs. At times reason does not prevail. It seems that there is more of a willingness to spend money and allocate resources for family disaster relief rather than family disaster prevention. The result is that "the void of need is too deep and the ladder of relief is too short." This is especially true for those families responsible for the primary caregiving of a family member during the home and community re-entry process when ideal aspirations are tempered by reality. This is most critical when a family member moves from the built-in respite care of a hospital, rehabilitation center, or nursing home and returns to the home or family environment.

Often a stark reality emerges when the family member arrives home and the basic equipment and supports, even if promised for the homecoming, are not in place. This is often a rude awakening that crystallizes what will actually be required to provide caregiving in the home. One way to avoid this situation or to minimize its impact is to have family members and caregivers be involved in self-help groups that prepare and support families in addressing and adjusting to these situations. The exposure to role models who have personal experiences and perspectives can be very helpful in exploring how other people cope with problems, navigate the health care system, and create solutions.

Addressing the importance of personal perspectives and experiences Armstrong (1991) stated:

> Without the day to day experience of the patient's irresponsibility, impulsivity, or other problems, or of the duties, other relatives can easily misperceive the caretaker as being too protective or restrictive, or too neglectful or uncaring. Examples of this are unending, and even those professionals who are most

committed or most caring can make these mistakes. Only those who have experienced the daily vigilances of care and worry are likely to be fully grateful and emotionally supportive of the family's accomplishments in fostering the patient's improvements (p. 20).

Personal experiences and perspective are also most relevant to those persons in need of home support related to palliative care. Costantini, Higginson, Boni, Orengo, Garone, Henriquet, & Bruzzi (2003) discussed the benefit of home care teams for the terminally ill:

One benefit of palliative home care teams is that they enable patients to remain at home for longer, by controlling symptoms and other problems and supporting the patient, family, and professionals (p. 315).

The key point is that while it is a noble goal to be at home at a time of great need, what can make a dramatic difference is the support of the family during this most demanding and potentially rewarding time. Often when a family is doing a great job the presumption is that they have all they need. While this may be true, it does not preclude further exploration of the situation and an evaluation of what may be needed in the future.

The following case indicates that even with adequate family resources to provide extraordinary care, the caregiving situation can become uniquely stressful and problematic.

Twelve children and their spouses were living within two miles of each other. The family consultant initially thought that designing and implementing a functional caregiving and respite-care intervention would be very possible given the number of family members and their combined resources. Unfortunately, the family relegated care to an unmarried daughter, who had health issues of her own, and their only participation was at a minimal and frequently critical level. The other children would insist that their mother, who had middle-stage Alzheimer's, receive the best care and only from the daughter, because no stranger should be allowed to take care of their mother. Regrettably and predictably, the primary caregiver became ill herself. The mother was placed in a nursing home and the family reached a state of dysfunction by not speaking to each other and blamed the caregiving sister because she became ill.

Quantitatively, this family had the structure and resources to provide an effective and efficient family-based caregiving and respite-care system. However, due to their inability to make the transition from a physically healthy family to a family with a sick parent, they were stuck at a level of disassociation due to a lack of commitment and a history of dysfunctional communication and interaction. Even when supportive services and other options were presented, they refused to accept them because it would increase their responsibility, even though it was a way for them to reduce chaos and to minimize dysfunction. But, as often occurs, some families are unable to mobilize their resources and do what may be in everyone's best interests, even when it is reasonable to do so.

WELLNESS: A COUNTERBALANCE TO STRESS IN CAREGIVING

When addressing the caregiver's health and wellness, the health professional may become aware that, in the process of adaptation to and coping with illness and disability, caregivers may tend to neglect themselves. Also, they may believe that the harder they work and the more they focus on those in need the more likely they will have an improved outcome. While this may happen sometimes, it is not always the case, and there are other issues to consider, as the following example demonstrates. When a young adult living with a severe disability was asked how she felt about her mother who took care of her for 25 years, she said that she was angry because her mother neglected herself and her father, and that was very distressing to her. She wished that there were more balance to her mother's life because she felt responsible for the mother's ill health because of the ongoing caregiving she provided. When this was discussed with the mother, she said, "I felt responsible for her condition and I thought that if I completely devoted myself to caregiving and did not take care of myself, I would feel better and be better able to cope. It did work some, but I wish I knew then what I know now."

Given the demands and toll of stress, the wellness and well-being of the caregiver should be given appropriate consideration. Berg-Weger, McGarthland-Rubio, and Tebb (2000) commented on the exploration of the well being of the caregiver as an important topic of consideration and investigation:

> Caregiver well-being is a relatively recent area of exploration for researchers and practitioners . . . Caregiver well-being should be considered in multidimensional terms . . . (p. 164).

Caregiver well-being and perception of burden are important issues because if the caregiver is overwhelmed by the demands of the caregiving process, it can result in caregiver burnout or caregiver role fatigue. In turn, this may create a situation where a potentially viable family home care situation is lost by default.

But social support can also be an invaluable resource contributing to caregiver well being.

In a discussion of social support in the context of emotional states and physical health, Salovey, Rothman, Detweiler, and Steward (2000) commented:

> Social supports may thus lead the individual to experience a lesser degree of stress in the face of a challenging situation. Social relationships may also allow individuals to feel secure with the knowledge that help will be provided when and if necessary(p. 116).

However, feeling secure in these situations may only last until the expectation of support is validated by it being there when needed. Addressing the differences in family coping and the importance of support in the prevention of additional negative consequences for both the family member and the caregiver, Levine, (2000) in her most timely book, *Always on Call*, stated that:

> Differences in family circumstances are critical factors in determining the level and kind of family responsibility that is both fair and achievable. Some families cope very well in exceptionally trying situations with little or no outside assistance. Others find the burdens overwhelming, resulting in sub-standard home care, potential abuse, neglect, and eventual institutionaliza-tion for the family member; poor health for the caregiver; and sometimes irrevocable family dissention and impoverishment (p. 12).

In some situations families may be willing to help out but their contributions may be more problematic than helpful. Grant, Ram-charan, McGrath, Holan, and Keady (1998) addressed the lack of family support and the problems related to it:

> First there were those who maintained a polite distance, but were clearly not available for practical helping purposes. Secondly, there were those whose help was an encumbrance and merely disabled caring efforts (p. 68).

These concerns are most understandable due the complexity of skills often required to be a caregiver, especially in very difficult situations. Often these situations require, if not demand, that the caregiver master not only physical challenges of basic activities of caregiving but also the complicated and emotionally stressful tasks related to the process of interacting and relying on family members. This can be most difficult when the behavior of the family member in need is not conducive to the caregiving process and is in effect detrimental to it.

MARITAL RELATIONSHIPS: IMPACT ON CAREGIVING

When the marriage ceremony includes the words "For better or worse, in sickness and in health" not everyone has the same understanding of what this means and what it could demand. Solid marital relationships can make the caregiving process and family life more reasonable. Kriegsman, Penninx, and vanEijk (1994) stated the importance of the marital relationship:

> The most important factor affecting the health of the family members is the quality of the marital relationship and, in particular, the amount of social support the patient is able to give the spouse (p. 249).

Knop, Bergman-Evans, and Warton-McCabe (1998) discuss the relationship between coping and the quality of marital relationships as they influence the caregiving process of spouses with Alzheimer's disease. The quality of the marital relationship has a role in determining how the caregiver will respond to the demands of the caregiving process (Morris, Morris, & Britton, 1988). In long-term care situations the caregiving burden can become more difficult because unresolved issues and marital discord intensify as the needs of the recipient of care increase (Wright, 1993). For example, an individual who values a quality relationship with his or her spouse may be better able to make the transition from marital partner to caregiver than someone who is in a toxic relationship and is looking for a way out, not a long-term commitment to a stressful caregiving role. This point is illustrated by a statement made to the authors by a friend who was asked how he was able to manage taking care of his wife with Alzheimer's as well as deal with his cancer. He stated, "She was a great wife once. She raised our children and took care of me when I was ill. I will be there as long as I can for her. I know she would do the same for me if she were capable."

Having a strong marriage or relationship is not a guarantee that the transition to caregiving will be successful. However, a solid relationship as well as a functional life and living perspective means that there is a greater probability that caregiving can be sustained. Under difficult circumstances, it is important to note that many solid relationships can be fractured while some marginal or problematic relationships can be refocused and enhanced by an illness or disability experience. Schultz and Quittner, (1998) addressed an important point when they commented on the reciprocal interaction between care recipient and caregiver:

> Caregiving, by definition, occurs in a social relational context. Yet little attention has been given to the reciprocal impact that patients and support persons have on each other (p. 110).

COMPENSATION IN CAREGIVING: FINANCIAL AND EMOTIONAL

In the current world of managed care and managed costs, some providers, administrators, policy makers, and others may expect that families will or should be in a position to assume more involved caregiving roles, often with little or no compensation, respite, or acknowledgement. This is presumptuous and potentially risky for all involved. Schultz and Quittner (1998) discuss the lack of compensation for caregiving as well as the limited alternatives to assuming this role:

> Although caregivers may perform tasks similar to those carried out by paid health professionals, they perform these services for no compensation and do so either voluntarily or because they feel there are no other alternatives(p. 107).

Focusing on what caregivers provide in unpaid services, Levine (1999) stated:

> Health care policy makers and analysts rarely consider the impact of these (financial) incentives on the 25 million unpaid, informal caregivers in the United States, who get little from the system in return for the estimated $196 billion a year in labor they provide (p. 1587).

This is most unfortunate because families are often forced, by default or intent, to provide what should be a basic and integral part of health and human care. An important question to address is how families can be supported and have access to those resources that acknowledge the value of their efforts, sacrifices, and significant contributions.

Levine (1999) also addressed the importance of caregiver support and the implications if it is lacking:

> Family caregivers must be supported, because the health care system cannot exist without them. Exhausted caregivers may become care recipients, leading to a further, often preventable, drain on resources (p. 1559).

This is a critical point because, without such support, individual family members or the family as a whole can be in a position of increased risk for burnout as well as behaviors that may increase the potential for additional problems. In effect a bad situation may get worse even if some help is available but is not worth the effort of accessing it.

RESPITE CARE

Respite care is often complementary and adjunctive to caregiving and can make a difference regarding the family's ability to sustain and maintain caregiving. This is most critical when the long-term issues related to chronic care are considered. Stober-Larsen (1998) commented on respite care programs as a response to distress:

> A recognition of the distress caregivers frequently experience has led to development of various services to support them, such as respite programs, hospice care, caregiver support groups, adult day care, in home help, and general psychosocial interventions (p. 26).

Just as there is variability in the populations served, there are differences in the definitions of respite care. Cohen and Warren (1985) provide the following:

> The definition of respite care as "the temporary care of a disabled individual for the purpose of providing relief to the primary caregiver" seems straightforward and non controversial. However, in practice, there is considerable variation in the interpretation of the scope of services to be called respite care. One of these variations concerns the distinction between intermittent and ongoing services. Virtually all definitions of respite care include the idea of temporary services (p. 26).

The problem with a time-limited definition of respite care is that the needs, problems, and concerns of both the patient and family may fluctuate and continue over a lifetime. This is especially true for the family of the person challenged by a complicated medical situation resulting in long-term needs and limited by short-term resources.

While the definitions of respite care focus upon the importance of providing relief for the family or caregiver, they also address the importance of relief by respite care. However, the presumption is often that support is available and accessible, but this is not always true.

Since illness and disability do not impact everyone at the same point in the same way during the life span, it is imperative that caregiving and respite care programs have the potential to respond to evolving and changing needs. While the nature of illness and disability plays a major role in the determination of need, consideration must also be given to the complexities of the emerging interaction between the family and the family member in need and the existence and accessibility of respite care programs. While family history, personal experiences, and role models can be important factors in creating the perspective needed to meet the demands of an illness and disability experience, the outcomes are not always ideal. For example, if the caring for a family member has created a significant amount of family stress, family members, individually or collectively, may decide that they will never again place themselves in a similar situation. However, some families may be able to recognize why the situation is or was so stressful and make changes and adaptations which can reduce stress and make the future situation more bearable, functional, and positive.

Even if the basic roles and functions of health care systems are distinct from those of the family, these systems should be complementary both to caregiving and respite care goals, and not adversarial to them. Unfortunately, most health care and political systems are burdened by policies and finances, while caregivers and consumers of respite care services are often more concerned with emotional survival and quality of life, often feeling the pressure to do more with less support. Addressing the need for family caregivers to set limits, Durgin (1989) stated:

> It is critical that family members be aware of their limitations and not feel pressured to take on too much responsibility. Typically, there are a large number of professionals involved in rehabilitation because it is too extreme a challenge for one to "shoulder it all." Families should be sure to say "no" when they cannot take on more and should also let it be known when they would like to be more involved (p. 22).

While recognizing the increased opportunities that have resulted from deinstitutionalization, Mesibov and Price (1995) pointed out that new problems and challenges for the community and family have been created. Families and caregivers often need their family member to have 24-hour care, and respite care is critical in helping families cope with the stress related to the often all-consuming caregiving process. The complexities of the problems have become a focal point for policy makers (Kane & Penrod, 1995) and caregivers are often lost or forgotten in the process (Levine, 1998, 1999; Houts, Nezu, Nezu, & Bucher, 1996).

Many family members may be able to tolerate a life of self-denial for a few days or weeks, but most won't be able to endure a regimen of

emotional and social deprivation indefinitely without becoming physically ill or emotionally wrought. For some families there are limited
options and they may be forced to provide caregiving roles for many
months, years, or even a lifetime.

The need for caregiving and respite care, therefore, is due to the
fact that families living with illness and or disability experiences are
often challenged by long-term situations, which may last a lifetime.
Acute illness has a built-in respite due to a time limitation imposed by
either death or substantial recovery, while chronic conditions have
expanding and long-term demands which can intensify the need for
sustained caregiving as well as respite care.

Not only does respite care help families cope with the challenges of
illness and disability, it helps the person affected by these conditions.
Their basic needs can be met by the respite care process and they are
afforded the chance for "nonmaintenance or nonconflictual interaction" with their families.

CONCLUSION

Effective, relevant, and accessible systems of caregiving and respite care
help families address and cope with the demands of the illness and
disability experience. There are few families who can make the transitions from wellness to state of loss, and respond constructively, if their
prior interactions have been problematic and dysfunctional. Families
who work together, who care about each other, and who have positive
and functional role models often make the adjustments that are supportive and helpful.

The need for caregiving and respite care emerges from the reality
that families living with illness and/or disability experiences are often
challenged by long-term situations that may last a lifetime. Acute illness
has a built-in respite due to a time limitation while chronic conditions
have expanding and long-term demands that can intensify the need
for sustained caregiving as well as respite care. Not only does respite
care help families cope with the challenges of illness and disability, but
also it helps persons impacted by these conditions. Their basic needs
can be met by the respite care process and they are afforded the chance
for "non-maintenance or non-conflictual interaction" with their families. The value of proactive caregiving and relevant respite care initiatives
is that they enable families to maximize their chances for survival when
challenged by illness and disability. Why should people, in extreme
need, feel neglected, abandoned and isolated? Can we not learn from

each other, share mutual strengths, and create an environment that facilitates, encourages, supports, and values caregiving and respite care values, programs and initiatives? Schultz and Quittner (1998) commented on the need to consider a broader caregiving and respite care perspective:

> Existing intervention studies have been either narrowly focused on a specific problem such as providing respite for the caregiver, or of the kitchen sink variety, where interventionists provide a little bit of everything. Neither approach has paid much attention to the articulation or measurement of mechanisms through which interventions might achieve their desire effects. This should receive high propriety in future studies (p. 110).

Illness and disability have the power to challenge the resources of the family as well as to create opportunities for new beginnings. Effective caregiving and accessible respite care have the potential to put illness, disability, aging, and other life changes into perspective and creates options so that families can live as fully as possible while creating positive and functional intergenerational legacies. Illness, disability and aging are not always traumas that negate humanity, but rather life experiences that gives people a chance to apply their values, as well as test their skills, while demonstrating how caring, committed and realistic they are. Though caregiving and respite care should be a component of a comprehensive intervention, treatment, health care and rehabilitation model, attention must be given to the multi-dimensional problems that families often face, such as role fatigue, stress, the need to rejuvenation, and the importance of maintaining quality of life.

The enormity of illness and disability is so pervasive that coping with it cannot be the sole responsibility of the family. Therefore, it is imperative that health care professionals be aware of the complexities surrounding the experience and how it has impacted the family in the past as well as the present and future.

Health care professionals have many different challenges when confronted with a family either deciding on respite care options or planning to provide some other form of caregiving assistance at home. This decision-making represents a vulnerable time for family members, since they will usually undergo some transition in family life and need to respond to new demands associated with the disability or chronic illness. The health care professional can provide both family support and gain an understanding of the specific issues prompted by respite care intervention. Also, the assessment model explained in Chapter 5 identifies many family areas that should be explored. During the family's transition to respite care, there are specific aspects of family life that need special assessment attention, such as particular stressors associated with the respite or extraordinary care decision, the identification of support resources, understanding the quality of family relationships, and the family member's willingness to take care of oneself while engaging in intensive caregiving responsibilities. Building on a family assessment, Chapter 6, *An Intervention Approach*, suggests many basic helping skills that can be utilized by the health care professional during respite care situations. Because respite care and long-term caregiving introduce several complexities for those who wish to provide assistance, many helping roles will be enacted during the intervention, including assessor, provider of support, and communication of needed information. Each role highlights the reality that caregiving has many dimensions, and interventions should be designed to meet the unique needs of individual families.

JUDY: MY MOTHER AND
AMYOTROPHIC LATERAL SCLEROSIS (ALS)

The following personal statement, related to a person with amyotrophic lateral sclerosis, addresses the importance of caregiving and respite care and captures many of the issues raised in this chapter. It reflects the journey of a very special lady as well as that of her daughter and family.

In the early spring, when the ground is soft, I will lay a marker on my mother's grave, a permanent marker to commemorate the life of a very special lady. The inscription will be short, impersonal, and incomplete—somehow not befitting a woman who courageously struggled against a devastating and cruel terminal illness. I cannot inscribe her story in stone, but I can set it on paper as a lasting tribute. I hope it will be a comfort to those who are afflicted with a serious or terminal illness, and a help to the families and health professionals who are involved in their care and treatment.

It was going to be an unbearably oppressive day, but my mother had no intention of sitting in her small, air-conditioned apartment. She set out early with her walking buddies on their five-mile jaunt and, as usual, took the lead. She was amused that her companions, who towered over her five-foot frame, could not keep up with her brisk pace. Everything seemed to be going well for her and my dad. Retirement for them was not a sedentary life, but rather one that was full and gratifying. In a few weeks, they would return to their apartment in Boston for five months of relief from Florida's intolerable heat.

But for now Betty was enjoying her walk and thinking about how rich her life was. As she turned the bend, her thoughts were interrupted abruptly by a stiffening of her left leg, perhaps a cramp, but she did not have the pain associated with a cramp. Her gait slowed considerably, and in a minute she found herself lying on her side. She was stunned by this unexpected interruption. She did not stumble over a rock or a crack in the roadside. What should she attribute this weakness to? It took five months for the doctors to make an accurate diagnosis. An electromyogram (EMG) was performed at the Brigham and Women's Hospital, and it was this test that ultimately determined that my mother had amyotrophic lateral sclerosis (ALS), commonly known as Lou Gehrig's disease, a progressive, degenerative disease that is terminal. It is probably the most dreaded neurological disease, and is one with no known cause or cure. Within one year of the first visible symptom, Betty would be a virtual paraplegic, confined to a wheelchair, unable to talk or to feed herself. Breathing and swallowing would become progressively more difficult. At no time would the disease affect her mental faculties, and she would always be aware of the creeping paralysis.

My initial reaction to the diagnosis was one of disbelief, devastation, and helplessness. How could such an active and health-conscious person be stricken with such a catastrophic illness? I felt a sadness for my parents, and I had real concerns about my dad's health also. It was conceivable to me that this tragedy could destroy him as well, and I prepared myself for the worst. The family and doctors were in total agreement as to how much to tell my mother. She had always been petrified of doctors and hospitals, and was by nature very nervous and anxious. We knew that she could not cope with such outrageous news. She was told that she had a chronic neuromuscular disease, and that she would need intensive therapy. We did not offer her hope of a cure, nor did we inform her that she was terminally ill. She asked very few questions, wanted to know as little as possible about her disease, and became adept at tuning out whatever she was not ready to hear.

Like my mother, my aunt, my father, and my brother went to great lengths to avoid the truth. Denial became a protective measure they would use effectively throughout the course of the illness. As much as I tried to beat through this barrier, I was met with resistance. It was this resistance that was to become a great source of frustration and anger for me. My aunt held out the longest, talking about the research, cures, and the possibility of people living several years. My brother, who never coped with adversity very well, did not become an integral part of the team, and his visits to the nursing home were often sporadic and brief. I had to know all the medical aspects of the disease, so I asked a lot of questions and read many books on ALS, and on death and dying. Someone had to take charge, to plan, and to carry the family through this crisis.

From the Brigham and Women's Hospital, my mother was transferred to the Braintree Rehabilitation Hospital. It was there that she was put on a daily regimen of physical, speech, and occupational therapies. She was extremely tense and frightened, but the staff was very professional and experienced, and knew how to respond to her emotional as well as physical needs. This was really not a time for rehabilitation as much as a time for enormous adjustment. It also allowed the family to make plans for home health care. I wished that my mother could stay at Braintree indefinitely, for I feared that the support systems at home would not be adequate. My fears were well founded. She was barely home two months when all the systems began to break down. My mother required constant attention and the Visiting Nurse's Association and private-home health professionals were not able to keep up with her demands. Oftentimes, my father was left without help, and he had to assume the role as primary caregiver. Tensions mounted and tempers began to flare, and what was once a very happy marriage now appeared to be very strained. My dad's health was deteriorating along with my mother's, and they looked to me for a quick solution. I knew that my mother required round-the-clock care in a skilled nursing facility, but I did not want to be responsible for initiating the search. I couldn't find it in my heart to do this to her, especially when she threatened to commit suicide before she would enter a nursing home. My grandmother had taken her own life because she could not cope with a painful illness, so I was worried about my mother's intentions. I began to get pressure from her sister, also, in defiance of any plan to move my mom from her home. We were in a crisis and we needed help quickly.

I was fortunate to find a psychologist who would help me accept and confront problems that were difficult and painful. He helped me see issues more clearly when everything seemed overwhelming and confusing; and it was through him that I began to understand the complexities surrounding chronic and terminal illnesses. His continued support and genuine concern were to sustain me through some very difficult times, the first of which was my mother's move to a nursing home. The transition from the apartment to the nursing home was traumatic for the family. Ostensibly, the home was attractive and meticulously maintained, with spacious rooms and beautiful furnishings. In sharp contrast to this orderliness was a picture of deterioration—of very old people in their eighties and nineties ravaged by debilitating disease, marked with permanent deformities, hooked up to life-support machines, and impaired by mental illness.There was also an aura of sadness and loneliness, and a sense that many of these people were deserted by their families.

I wished that I could put blinders on my mother's eyes, to shut out a world that was so unreal, yet only too real and disheartening. My mother was only 69 years old and looked ten years younger. How could we do this to her! I knew that there was no alternative, but I was stricken with guilt, a guilt that was to stay with me for a long time. It took a good three months before I could walk into the nursing home without feeling sick, without feeling very, very shaken.

I don't think my mother ever adjusted to nursing home life. I think she resigned herself to her fate. I know she often felt very sad, lonely, and misunderstood, but I do not think she felt abandoned. She knew that the family was there for her, and it was this prevailing sense of security that kept her from slipping into a deep depression. A schedule was worked out so that one or two family member would visit daily. This was arranged mostly out of love, partly out of guilt, and out of an acute awareness that strangers would not minister to her needs the way family would. We also knew that if we were

going to survive this ordeal we would have to share the responsibilities, for
each of us had a history of medical problems. Often the burden of responsibility rested on my shoulders, and at times I felt overwhelmed. But I also felt
that if my mother could cope with the effects of a very disabling disease, I
could deal with any problems that arose.

I do not know how she endured all the suffering, and I do not understand
what held her together. She certainly did not triumph over her disease—she
did not write a book, or paint by mouth, or engage in anything that was
extraordinary. She just tried to get through the day. There were many tears
and many moments of anguish, but even in her despair she insisted on getting
up, getting dressed, and above all, having her hair done weekly. Thank God
there was a hairdresser on the premises, and thank God she still cared about
her appearance. Throughout her illness, she never lost her sense of humor
or her ability to smile and laugh. But the laughing was done for the staff,
and most of the crying was done with the family. We tried to maintain a sense
of equilibrium, but it was difficult to keep control when all systems were
failing. The disease was progressing at an alarming rate, and we knew she
would need the strong support of the family and the specialized services of
many health care professionals. Some services were effective, but most fell
short. Many professionals were not familiar with or could not cope with the
demands of ALS. They were uneasy in treating a terminally ill patient, or
clearly had an attitude problem toward the sick and the elderly. I must
acknowledge, though, that most people did try to help, and I cannot fault
them for their human limitations in dealing with a very difficult case. I also
believe that my mother's inability to speak had a lot to do with the quality
of care she received. This was a great source of frustration for her as well as
for the health professionals who worked with her. The family members were
the only ones who had the patience to make use of the communication boards.
We acted as liaison between my mother and the staff, so our involvement in
her care was crucial.

We also acted as her advocates and protectors. There were aspects of
nursing home care that were unsettling, but because we had a very good
working relationship with the staff, most of our grievances were worked out.
I can only think of one incident that was offensive and repulsive, and it was
due to a personality conflict between my mother and an aide. An aide had
lost control and, out of anger and impatience, threw a sheet over my mother's
head. This was a gross violation of my mother's right to be treated as a living
human being until the day she died.

The issue of support systems was always a source of great pain and anguish
for me. My anxiety was heightened by my mother's refusal to discuss these
matters and the inability of family members to agree on a specific course of
action. I personally believed that the use of heroic measures, in my mother's
case, would be cruel and inhumane—a prolongation of inexorable suffering
pain and an interference with the natural order of things. But I had to know
where my mother stood on these issues for, ultimately, it was her life and
her decision. Three months before her death, she began to make her wishes
known. She slowly spelled out the word *die* every day. She made it quite clear

to me that she could no longer tolerate living. She finally came to terms with her death, knew it was imminent, and had an urgency to express her grief and fears about dying. Once she accepted her death, she became more tranquil. I did not want my mother to die in the arms of strangers, nor did I want her to experience death alone. I was fortunate to be with her at the moment of death. My aunt and I sat by her side and held her hands, and except for a brief interruption by staff, this was a family affair. We exchanged a few words of support and comfort, but we were mostly caught up in remembering and recollecting. I wondered if my mother saw her life flashing before her, and if she were passing through the dark tunnel toward Omega, but I could not be sure.

DISCUSSION QUESTIONS

1. How do family values and traditions influence the caregiving process?
2. Why was the nursing home placement stressful for this family?
3. What were the issues for Judy's father?
4. Do you think it would be important for all family members to take a more supportive role in the caregiving process? How can this happen?
5. Would you respond differently if your spouse had ALS?

SET 10: HOW CAN I HELP?

PERSPECTIVE

A characteristic of most suffering is that it is done alone. This is especially true when families are forced to retreat from society and focus all of their energy on the caregiving process. A major tenet of respite care is that the more a burden is shared, the more bearable it becomes.

EXPLORATION

1. Do you know a family dealing with a disability? With ALS? Have you considered reaching out and providing support?
2. Would you respond differently if the person with ALS were your mother or father?
3. How would the experience of Alzheimer's disease differ from that of ALS?

4.   If you belong to a religious organization, can you identify how this religious organization demonstrates the principle of becoming involved like "the good Samaritan" by taking care of people in this life as well as the next?

REFERENCES

Angell, M. (1999). The American health care system revisited: A new series, *New England Journal of Medicine, 340*, 48.

Armstrong, C. (1991). Emotional changes following brain injury: Psychological and neurological components of depression, denial and anxiety. *Journa. of Rehabilitation,* June, 14–17.

Arno, P., Levine, C., & Memmott, M., (1999). The economic value of informal caregiving. *Health Affairs, 18*(2), 182–188.

Bakas, T., & Burgener, S. C. (2002). Predictors of emotional distress, general health, and caregiving outcomes in family caregivers of strokesurvivors. *Topics in Stroke Rehabilitation, 9*(1), 34–45.

Berg-Weger, M., McGarthland-Rubio, D., & Tebb, S. S. (2000). Depression as a mediator: Viewing caregiver well-being and strain in a different light. *Families in Society, 81*(2), 162–173.

Biegel, D. E. (1995). Caregiving. In A. E. Dell Orto & R. P. Marinelli (Eds.), Encyclopedia of Disability and Rehabilitation. New York: Simon & Schuster/ Macmillan.

Brandstater, M. E., & Shutter, L. A. (2002). Rehabilitation interventions during acute care of stroke patients. *Topics in Stroke Rehabilitation, 9*(2), 48–56.

Brandt, A. L. (1998). *Caregiver's reprieve.* San Luis Obispo, CA: Impact Publishers.

Breckbill, J., & Carmen, S. (1999). Support for families and children with special needs. *Caring, 18*(2), 6–10. Christensen, K. A., Stephens, M. A., & Townsend, A. L. (1998). Mastery in women's multiple roles and well-being: Adult daughters providing care to impaired parents. *Health Psychology, 17,* 163–171.

Christensen, K. A., Stephens, M. A., & Townsend, A. L. (1998). Mastery in women's multiple roles and well-being: Adult daughters providing care to impaired parents. *Health Psychology, 17,* 163–171.

Cocks, A. (2000). Respite care for disabled children: Micro and macro reflections. *Disability & Society, V15, N3,* 507–519.

Cohen, S., & Warren, R. (1985). *Respite care.* Austin, TX: Pro Ed.

Costantini, M., Higginson, I., Boni, L., Orengo, M. A., Garone, E., Henriquet, F., & Bruzzi, P. (2003). Effect of a palliative home care team on hospital admissions among patients with advanced cancer. *Palliative Medicine, 17,* 315–321.

D'Asaro, A. (1998). Caring for yourself is caring for your family: Methods of coping with the everyday stresses of caregiving. *Exceptional Parent, 28*(6), 38–40.

Dell Orto, A.E., & Power, P.W. (2000). *Brain injury and the family: A life and living perspective.* (2nd ed.) Boca Raton, FL: CRC Press.

Dowling, M., & Dolan, L. (2001). Families with children with disabilities:Inequalities and the social model. *Disability & Society, 16*(1), 21–35.

Durgin, C. J. (1989). Techniques for families to increase their involvement in the rehabilitation process. *Cognitive Rehabilitation,* May/June, 22–25.

Eaves, Y. D. (2002). Rural African American caregivers' and stroke survivors' satisfaction with health care. *Topics in Geriatric Rehabilitation, 17*(3), 72–84.

Ergh, T. C., Rapport, L. J., Coleman, R. D., & Hanks, R. (2002). A Predictor of caregiver and family functioning following traumatic brain injury: Social support moderates caregiver distress. *Journal of Head Trauma Rehabilitation, 17*(2), 155–174.

Fredriksen, K.I., & Scharlach, A.E. (1999). Employee family care responsibilities. *Family Relations,* 48, 189-196.

Gardner, W. (2002). The impact of behavior problems on caregivers after traumatic brain injury. *Brain Injury Source,* 6,1, winter, 40-43.

Gillen, R., Tennen, H., Affleck, G., & Steinpreis, R. (1998). Distress, depressive symtoms, and depressive disorder among caregivers of patients with brain injury. *Journal of Head Trauma Rehabilitation, 13*(3), 31–43.

Grant, G., Ramcharan, P., McGrath, M., Holan, M., & Keady, J. (1998). Rewards and gratifications among family caregivers: Toward a refined model of caring and coping. *Journal of Intellectual Disability Research, 42*(1), 58–71.

Hartke, R. J., & King, R. B. (2002). Analysis of problem types and difficulty among older stroke caregivers. *Topics in Stroke Rehabilitation, 9*(1), 16–33.

Hecht, M. J., Graesel, E., Tigges, S., Hillemacher, T., Winterholler, M., Hilz, M. J., Heuss, D., & Neundo, B. (2003). Burden of care in amyotrophic lateral sclerosis. *Palliative Medicine, 17,* 327 333.

Houts, P., Nezu, A., Nezu, C., & Bucher, J. (1996). The prepared family caregiver: A problem solving approach to family caregiving education. *Patient Education and Counseling, 27,* 63–73.

Jarman, D. J., & Stone, J. A. (1989). Brain injury: issues and benefits arising with a family support group. *Cognitive Rehabilitation,* May/June, 30–32.

Kahana, E., Biegel, D. F., & Wykle, M. L., Eds. (1994). *Family caregiving across the life span.* Newbury Park, CA: Sage.

Kane, R., & Penrod, J. (1995). *Family caregiving in an aging society: Policy erspectives.* Thousand Oaks, CA: Sage Publications.

Knop, D. S., Bergman-Evans, B., & Warton-McCabe, B. (1998). In sickness and in health: An exploration of the perceived quality of the marital relationship, coping, and depression in caregivers of spouses with Alzheimer's disease. *Journal of Psychosocial Nursing, 36*(1), 16–21.

Kosciulek, J., & Lustig, D. (1998). Predicting family adaptation from brain injury:Related family stress. *Journal of Applied Rehabilitation Counseling, 29*(1), 8–12.

Kramer, B., (2000). Husbands caring for wives with dementia. *Health and Social Work, 25*(2), 97–107.

Kriegsman, D. M., Penninx, B. W., & vanEijk, J. T. (1994). Chronic disease in the elderly and its impact on the family: a review of the literature. *Family Systems Medicine, 12*(3), 249–267.

Kriegsman, D. M., Penninx, B. W., & vanEijk, J. T. (1995). A criterion-based literature survey of the relationship between family support and incidence and course of chronic disease in the elderly. *Family Systems Medicine, 13*(1), 39–68.

Levine, C. (Ed.) (2000). *Always on Call. New York:* United Hospital Fund.

Levine, C. (1999). The loneliness of the long-term caregiver. *The New England Journal of Medicine, 340*(20), 1587–1590.

Levine, C. (1998). *Rough crossings: Family caregivers' odysseys through the health care system.* New York: United Hospital Fund

Lustig, D. (1999). Family caregiving of adults with mental retardation: Key issues for rehabilitation. *Journal of Rehabilitation, 65*(2), 26–35.

McGrath, W. L., Mueller, M. M. Brown, C., Teitelman, J., & Watts, J. (2000). Caregivers of persons with Alzheimer's disease: An exploratory study of occupational performance and respite. *Physical and Occupational Therapy in Geriatrics, 18*(2), 51–69.

Mesibov, G. B., & Price, J. C. (1995). Respite care. In A. E. Dell Orto & R. P. Marinelli (Eds.), *Encyclopedia of Disability and Rehabilitation.* New York: Simon & Schuster/Macmillan.

Morris, R. G., Morris, L. W., & Britton, P. G. (1988). Factors affecting the emotional well being of the caregivers of dementia sufferers. *British Journal of Psychiatry, 153*, 147–156.

Newsom, J. T., & Schulz, R., (1998). Caregiving from the recipient's perspective: Negative reactions to being helped. *Health psychology, 17*, 172–181.

Power, P. W., Dell Orto, A. E.,& Gibbons, M.(1988). *Family interventions throughout illness and disability.* New York: Springer Publishing.

Salovey, P., Rothman, A. J., Detweiler, J. B., & Steward, W. T. (2000). Emotional states and physical health. *American Psychologist, 55*(1), 110–121.

Sander, A. M., Sherer, M., Malec, J. F., High, W. M., Thompson, R. N., Moessner, A. M., & Josey, J. (2003) Pre-injury emotional and family functioning in caregivers of persons with traumatic brain injury. *Archives of Physical Medicine and Rehabilitation, 84*(2), 197–203.

Schultz, R., & Quittner, A. L.,(1998). Caregiving for children and adults with chronic conditions: Introduction to the special issue, *Health Psychology, 17*(2), 107–111.

Shannon, J. B. (2001) *Caregiving sourcebook,* 1st ed. Detroit, MI: Omnigraphics.

Smith, J. E.,& Smith, D. L. (2000). No map, no guide: Family caregivers on their journeys through the system. *Care Management Journals, 2*(1), 27–33.

Stober-Larsen, L. (1998). Effectiveness of a counseling intervention to assist family caregivers of chronically ill relatives. *Journal of Psychosocial Nursing, 36*(8), 26–32.

Wright, L. K. (1993). Alzheimer's disease and marriage: An intimate account. Newbury Park, CA: Sage Publications.

Yee, J. L., & Schulz, R. (2000). Gender differences in psychiatric morbidity among family caregivers: A review and analysis. *The Gerontologist, 40*(2), 147–164.

Zeigler, E. A. (1989). The importance of mutual support for spouses of brain injury survivors. *Cognitive Rehabilitation,* May/June, 34–37.

11

Loss, Grief, and Grieving: Family Issues

INTRODUCTION

The diagnosis of an illness, acute, chronic, or terminal, as well as a severe disability can create, contribute to, or intensify a crisis in family life. It may also cause a family to enter a state of loss and subsequent grief that is intense, consuming, and enduring. Grief itself is a complex interaction of emotional, cognitive, spiritual, physiological, and behavioral responses to a situation of significant loss (Romanoff, 1993). It is the individual experience of the pain of loss (Kane, 1990). When a family is suddenly or gradually affected by a severe medical event, feelings of depression, resentment, anger, sadness, and grief emerge. These emotions also frequently emerge from cumulative illness/disability-related losses that are magnified or intensified by a current crisis in family life. It is important to understand, therefore, the issues related to loss and grief as part of the rehabilitation and health care process (Fell, 1994; Bowlby, 1980; Doka, 1995).

When unpredictable and even predictable events occur during the course of the treatment and rehabilitation process, the renewed feelings of loss and the accompanying pain of grief can interfere with coping, personal and family management, and the overall adaptive processes. To be noted is that grief is an emotion, whereas grieving is a coping process (Attig, 1996). Moreover, the causes and effects of grief are intertwined with complicated family dynamics. Many of the factors associated with health problems have been studied under the lens of family losses. Knowledge of family losses can pinpoint family needs and expectations. In their review of the literature, Lyons and Sullivan (1998) have identified three major approaches to understanding loss. The individual perspective has explored the assessment of illness-related stressors and how distressed family members can cope more productively with illness, disability, and other losses and changes in their lives. The social change perspective views loss as primarily caused by the social construction of illness and disability, and targets the need to change services, policies, and societal values. The relationship perspective maintains that social support is a key factor in managing and adapting to loss. Providing emotional and instrumental support to persons experiencing the grieving process is an important intervention strategy from the relationship perspective.

All these perspectives will be included in this chapter, since the reactions to loss and grief are influenced by a number of factors (Parkes, 1975; Pollock, 1961; Garner, 1997), and helping approaches to manage and even resolve grief must be developed in harmony with the myriad influences on family members of grief reactions. Although previous chapters in this book have discussed the many emotional reactions to chronic illness and severe disability, with the reality of loss a recurrent theme to the reactive experience, the causes and expressions of grief can be distinctive. Grieving usually demands specific adaptive skills, often has its own reactive time framework, and frequently necessitates for its management an internalized locus of control (Kane, 1990). Because loss and grief management require different intervention strategies, this chapter will emphasize such topics as 1) general considerations to identify when working with a family's loss and grief issues, 2) obstacles to effective grieving, and 3) grief responses by family members, including the identification of those influences on the grieving process. This material serves as a foundation for discussing interventions focused on meeting the family's current and future needs.

GENERAL CONSIDERATIONS

Before intervention approaches can be developed, health care professionals should have an understanding of those realities that will facilitate a helping strategy that is relevant to the family living with a chronic illness or severe disability.

UNDERSTANDING THE GRIEVING PROCESS

Grief responses by family members include emotions, thoughts, and behaviors that occur as a reaction to perceived family losses (Kane, 1990). Many losses are significant because of their symbolic meaning to the family (Brown, 1990). The perception of the importance of what has been lost affects the intensity and the duration of the grief. While grief is a normal and healthy reaction to loss, the strength and the duration of the family's grieving response is often unpredictable due to a variety of life stressors, some known and others not anticipated. When unanticipated or even predictable events occur, they can complicate the grieving process by forcing the family to fight several battles concurrently. Further complicating the grieving process are children's reactions to serious loss or death, which include fear, guilt, anger, and confusion (Wright & Oliver, 1993). These are all intense emotions that can create added distress both for children and for families because they may be feeling helpless to relieve the pain, replace the loss, or accelerate the mourning process.

Kane (1990) identifies a four-stage process of grief as a response to loss. In Kane's theory, grief resolution is an unchanging succession of stages: 1) ignoring the loss; 2) experiencing the loss; 3) understanding the loss; and 4) changing with the loss. When family members deny the loss, are evasive in their communication, show an absence of basic self-care and nurturing, and have persistent anger, guilt, hopelessness, and depression, they are displaying major adjustment problems. These will exact a toll over time and if not resolved may result in more difficulties and problems. This is often the case when families are so consumed by the crisis at hand that they are not vigilant, and consequently other problems and crises may occur which could have been anticipated or even prevented.

In contrast, the family that expresses an appropriate reactive sadness and begins to confront the reality of the loss and emerging, potential opportunities may be better able to meet its responsibilities. Family communication styles are still intact. There may be some regression by family members to more childish, aggressive behaviors, but it is often temporary. Their sadness is actually a necessary part of the grieving process, and the help provided to the family is mainly directed toward providing support for them.

Matz (1978) developed a lengthier descriptive model that captures many of the family's behavioral reactions, although families differ in how they react to the loss. Matz believes that there are different stages of mourning in response to a traumatic event, and if a bereaved family is to reach an adaptive stage, family members will usually follow predictable steps in their grieving processes:

1. "If I deny it, it's not true." The first response to a serious loss is usually denial, although Matz believes that the denial stage is "punctu-

ated" by times of painful emotional awareness. The denial helps the family members to function and to meet many of their daily responsibilities.

2. "I have the power to undo it." The denial gradually gives sway to feelings of omnipotence. These feelings may be characterized by attempting to bring back the loss by searching efforts, or it may be expressed as anger at events or people the bereaved family regards as responsible for the loss. Unfortunately these efforts are doomed to fail, and gradually despair and helplessness occur.

3. "I can't do anything about it." Matz explains this as a time when the bereaved family members face the loss and begin to understand their feelings in order to reach an adaptive solution. The past may be re-examined, perhaps given up, and partially replaced with hope. Depression also occurs, but hope may overcome it.

4. "I am rebuilding and every now and then I remember." The bereaved family members start to rebuild their lives. Social patterns are reestablished and new decisions are made to reach personal and family goals. According to Matz, painful memories will arise but the family members appear to have more strength to deal with these emotions.

With all of these steps, however, the phases do not have clear-cut beginnings and endings. The move from phase to phase is gradual rather than sudden and dramatic. Other stage models have been proposed, with the language differing from model to model (Bader & Robbins, 2001). Many of the published reactive grieving models have as a basic assumption that "grieving progresses from a state of initial numbness; through a stage of high arousal and distress characterized by pining and 'waves' of grief; ending in a resolution of grief . . . progress through the stages is facilitated by 'grief work' (Romanoff, 1993, p. 385).

The stages of grief, however, do not explain the intensity and differential expressions experienced by family members. Although recognition of the stages is useful (Davis, 1987), the linear sequence of stages commonly proposed by most theorists does not reflect the complexity of the adjustment process, particularly in those families experiencing chronic illness and severe disability. No data has been presented to date to demonstrate the reliability and validity of the sequence and duration of the reported stages, and there is little evidence that certain phases (e.g., denial, depression) are frequent responses to loss. The adaptive process to loss and grief is actually dependent on the nature of the crisis, triggering events, and contextual variables (Livneh & Antonak, 1997).

Understanding the Concepts of Centrality, Peripheral, Preventable, and Unpreventable

Bugen (1977) explains the meaning of these terms as follows: if the person is central to family life, such as a loving parent or successful child, the loss will be greater than that associated with a person who is peripheral to the family. Whether the trauma was preventable or unpreventable will influence anger and blame associated with the intensity of the loss response. These concepts are important to understand because the health care professional frequently assists the family to move from a belief in preventability to a belief in unpreventability. To be noted is that many disabilities are caused by the decisions, choices, action, or inaction of family members, friends, significant others, and strangers. For example, many parents are burdened with the reality that they bought the bicycle (with or without a helmet) or car (with or without airbags) that was related to the disability of their family member. If the person is central and the family members are convinced the injury was preventable, then as Bugen states, the grief will be both intense and prolonged. Initial intervention with the family will entail an assessment of the relationship of the impact of chronic illness/disability to the expectations, values, and beliefs of the family members.

Often those family members who reasonably adjust to the loss do so by drawing upon their resources and finding new meaning in living in spite of their family structure, dreams, and resources being greatly altered. Rolland (1994) compares second-order changes, which are "the altering aspects of one's world view and the basic rules that go with them" (p. 25), to first-order changes which are the intensification of efforts within the boundaries of traditional roles such as gender roles. But reconceptualizing the needs of caregivers as involving losses that need to be grieved rather than just solved by general support or specific information represents an important change in direction (Walker & Pomeroy, 1996). This is a significant development in grief and loss resolution because it attends to the depth of the issue rather than focusing on surface manifestations.

Flexibility of Intervention Goals for the Family Experiencing Loss and Intense Grieving

Families who are experiencing a chronic illness or disability will have different needs. Many family members are looking for alleviation of the feelings of loneliness, isolation, and depression, whereas others are searching for a way to integrate the loss into family life. The challenge for families is to accept the loss, adapt to the loss, and try to assimilate the chronic sorrow into the family system. Stroebe, Gergen, Gergen, and Stroebe (1992) emphasize the need to let go in order to move on:

> It might prove desirable to teach clients that there are many goals that can be set, many ways to feel and not a set series of stages that they must pass through—that many forms of expression and behavioral patterns are accept- able reactions to loss (p. 1221).

Kane (1990) emphasized that readjustment to loss and the achieve- ment of positive change are dependent on coping capabilities, the family members' flexibility and adaptability, internalized locus of control, and adaptive skills. For the family expressing grief, intervention efforts are not only directed to alleviating the immediate pain but also to increasing the ability of the family member to change appropriately and cope effectively with a permanent loss. Putting this in perspective, Stroebe, Gergen, Gergen, and Stroebe (1992) state:

> Grieving, a debilitating emotional response, is seen as a troublesome interfer- ence with daily routines, and should be 'worked through.' Such grief work typically consists of a number of tasks that have to be confronted and systemati- cally attended to before normality is reinstated (p. 1205).

This is not an easy or simple processes. In effect, families are often expected to deconstruct their world and redefine themselves in order to create a sense of purpose and meaning in their lives. The intensity of this process for caregivers living with multiple losses has been de- scribed as "the funeral that never ends" (Kapust & Weintraub, 1984, p. 462). However, the common reality we all share is that certain events of the life experience must be accepted for what they are, and they are not always amenable to being molded into what we want and need them to be.

ETHNIC AND GENDER DIFFERENCES IN EXPRESSING LOSS AND GRIEF

What is ethnically normal for one family may be unusual for another. The manner and length of time assumed normal for grieving differs greatly from culture to culture. In certain Mediterranean countries, such as Greece and Italy, for example, women have traditionally worn black for the rest of their lives after a husband's death . . . Cultures even differ in major ways about public versus private expressions of grief" (McGoldrick, et al., 1991, pp. 177–178). In many Hispanic cultures, women in particular are expected to express their sorrow dramatically, while in southeast Asian societies men and women are expected to be composed and stoical about their feelings (Osterweis, Solomon, & Green, 1984).

Individuals from varied cultures also view the world in differing ways. World view includes beliefs, values, and language, and they can affect a family member's performance in how he/she handles a significant loss and the resultant grieving (Whiston, 2000). Because of a lack of knowledge of gender and ethnic differences, there may be intolerance for the way another person or another ethnic family grieves. In fact, cultural differences may make one person's grieving seem bizarre to the other. It is important, therefore, for health care professionals to show respect for the cultural heritage and values of the family, especially when considering the timing for dealing with the emotional aftermath of a loss (McGoldrick, et al., 1991).

OBSTACLES TO PROGRESS IN GRIEVING

There are specific roadblocks to effective grieving, and from the authors' experience four have been identified.

A. *Persistent denial of the permanence of specific cognitive and physical losses.* Family members may continuously discuss "what was," and the past is repeatedly reviewed or dwelled upon in order to maintain hope for full recovery and restoration of function. Although the topics of death and dying are usually associated with bereavement, chronic illness and severe disability are events that can cause intense family grief because they cause a pervasive sense of change, finality, and loss. Many family members may refuse to accept a loss as real. This refusal "may be embedded in a more encompassing refusal to acknowledge and accept limitation, vulnerability, and powerlessness" (Attig, 1996, p. 40).

Zemzars (1984) stated that for all chronic illnesses, the person can never fully return to a pre-illness state of health. This does not mean that gains cannot be made or goals attained; it does mean that in life, time cannot be stopped. Each day brings change, and in that process there is a degree of irretrievable loss. This is due to the life-altering impact of events that transform the physical, emotional, and spiritual domains of family life.

The family's eventual realization that they and the family member will never be exactly the same can cause lingering feelings of deep sorrow. Miller, Houston, and Goodman (1994) reported that "losses suffered by the debilitating effects of head injuries, stroke, or central nervous system dysfunction can be conceptualized as a partial death" (p. 50).

B.   *Inability to express negative effect because of the loss.* Bowlby (1980) explains that anger and crying are necessary responses, which can lead to the recognition that the loss is final. The inability to cry or rave at the loss is often a consequence of society's dictates to maintain appropriate composure at the time of the loss. The initial grief response may also be inhibited because of a family member's fear of how a grief reaction may affect the injured family member or other members. Some families believe that the recognition or release of angry feelings associated with a loss is inappropriate. Also, a family member may be confused about the nature of his or her feelings about what has occurred. Self-blame or guilt may inhibit the expression of anger. Resentment about the implications of the loss for future planning may be personally perceived as inappropriate, thwarting any behaviors that might release the tension and grief caused by the loss.

C.   *Difficulties in dealing with ambivalence.* When the loss is uncertain it may be difficult to bring grief to a satisfactory conclusion. The course of a chronic illness may be uncertain, and a hope that is based on assumptions may inhibit a family member from coming to terms with a loss. Or, a family member may be physically present but psychologically "dead," e.g., deteriorating Alzheimer's individuals. Related to ambivalence is that the specific loss makes no sense. The question "Why did this happen to us?" triggers a constant, nagging search for explanation. This indefiniteness and search may prevent a family member from confronting the reality of what really has happened and delay the process of "letting go," which is essential for an eventual, adaptive, grieving process.

D.   *Unfinished business related to other losses.* All family members have a certain amount of "emotional baggage" which lingers in their life, but which may become quite expressive by a sudden, unexpected diagnosis or occurrence of a severe disability. Past losses may never have been completely resolved, discussed, or understood. The emotions of anger, hostility, self-blame, and guilt may still be festering, but are suppressed because of certain rules and demands of family life. The lack of resolution of previous losses or unresolved grief becomes a barrier for dealing with new separations and disappointments. The individual brings to coping efforts a double burden—lingering emotions that have a troubling effect on one's mental health, and the challenge to deal with a new, serious loss. Of particular interest is the influence of early parental loss on the development of subsequent complicated grief reactions (Worden, 1991).

FACTORS INFLUENCING THE GRIEVING PROCESS

There are several determinants to how a family will handle loss and subsequent grief precipitated by a member's chronic illness or severe disability. Many of these determinants are similar to the individual's reaction to the medical event, discussed in Chapter 3. One particular determinant identified earlier, but which receives a special emphasis related to intense loss, is who in the family has the chronic illness or severe disability. For example, the sorrow accompanying the severe illness/disability of a child is a profound, recurrent, cyclic sadness and is not confined to a time-bound process (Davis, 1987). The experience of intense sorrow can represent a continued grieving process. The factual loss may never become a significant memory, and the grieving process is never completed (Weisman, 1973). Other determinants, such as one's self-concept, a family's belief system, sociocultural context, gender differences, the presence or absence of a social support network, the stigma attached to the medical event (e.g., AIDS, suicide attempts, mental illness), and the lack of developed coping skills need to be re-emphasized when exploring the cause of difficulties in grieving or when planning intervention approaches.

Another determinant of particular significance is the life-cycle timing of loss. Untimely losses and those that concur with multiple losses or with other major family stresses may place a family at higher risk for dysfunctional consequences. A life-threatening injury or illness to a child, for example, may reverse generational expectations. The concurrence of a loss with other developmental milestones, such as a new marriage or the birth of a child may pose challenging tasks and demands. Also, a multigenerational family legacy of loss may leave family members more vulnerable to subsequent losses (Walsh & McGoldrick, 1991).

As identified earlier in this chapter, moreover, a relationship perspective is currently the focus of study when developing intervention approaches. The quality of a family relationship can be a key determinant in recognizing how an individual is managing the grieving process. With changes in health care and greater reliance on the family, the need for positive, family support has become more critical (Lyons & Sullivan,

1998). Reducing relationship tensions and exploring with the family mutually enjoyable activities may be an important ingredient in successful grieving adjustment. Although relationship stresses exist across a broad range of health problems and disabilities and are present in activities of work, leisure, intimacy, and social support, focusing on the nature of family relationships can contribute to valuable insights when developing intervention strategies to resolve intense grieving (Lyons & Sullivan, 1998).

FAMILY MEMBER RESPONSES TO LOSS AND SUBSEQUENT GRIEVING PATTERNS

The particular reaction of family members to a chronic illness or severe disability can differ within the same family. The timing of the grieving may also differ. Further, the type of response, e.g., sadness, anger, guilt, reproach, anxiety, loneliness, fatigue, and helplessness identified in earlier chapters may be the same because illness and disability usually means challenging losses. But with certain family members, such as parents or principal caregivers of young children, reactive emotions may be intensified, exaggerated, and lengthened (Worden, 1991; Power & Dell Orto, 2003). Despair, confusion, and yearning may accompany these emotions. The shock and severity of the illness or disability may leave parents feeling completely helpless. They may also find it very difficult to focus, since preoccupation to what has happened to the child may make it impossible to concentrate.

Worden (1991) believes that at the time of illness or disability onset, certain feelings, e.g., shock, denial, helplessness, may be overwhelming and may cause family members to delay their grief. Later events, such as leaving the hospital, or watching a film, television, or some other media event in which loss is the main theme may then stimulate those feelings, which have been lingering since disease or disability onset. What identifies the delayed grief reaction is the intensity of the feelings experienced by the family member, suggesting that the grief experience from earlier events is still unresolved.

GRIEF RESOLUTIONS: INTERVENTIONS

Intervention approaches have been discussed in chapter 6. Yet there are several differences from those strategies presented earlier when there is the intervention task of helping a family come to terms with the losses emerging from chronic illness and disability and then assisting family members to manage the accompanying grieving process. The losses themselves and dealing with personal grieving issues could be additional factors for family members to cope with when they are involved with their own adaptive concerns and, perhaps at the same time, assisting their family members with care giving needs during the treatment and rehabilitation process.

There are usually two differences from the intervention models proposed in chapter 6 when the health care professional also focuses specifically on the loss and grieving reactions of family members. One is the time factor. Earlier intervention strategies described approaches that would help the family "put into place" management responsibilities for their own and their family member's adjustment. Current tasks receive the focus of attention. The past must be put aside if caregiving is going to be helpful. Two previously identified "critical points" noted in Chapter 6 have passed, and the family is trying to live adaptively in face of the chronic illness/severe disability experience. But the process of grieving can last for years, with each new season or holiday providing the old sense of loss (McGoldrick, 1991). Even as treatment and rehabilitation efforts continue, family members often are still adjusting themselves to necessary changes and perhaps the absences of past satisfactions. Grieving may never be totally over, though eventually there comes a time when most families have in a general way adapted to the loss (McGoldrick, 1991).

Issues around the past have a dominant role in grief resolution. Instead of only attending to present tasks and challenges related to the family's adjustment, there is a need to reflect on past events contributing to the loss experience and past coping skills. How an individual adapts after loss is generally determined both by a review of past events and by his or her individual coping skills. Matz (1978) has identified these goals as the determinants of successful grief resolution. The family must become aware of the basic source of the loss because what may be perceived by the health care professional as the cause of family grief may only be another symptom of a more serious problem. For example, the occurrence of another disability for a parent who has a long family history of alcoholism and absence from home for prolonged periods may renew feelings or resentment, especially if that person has undergone alcoholism rehabilitation before the diagnosis. Family members may still harbor deep emotions about the patient's earlier behavior. This represents unfinished business, and the new diagnosis aggravates these feelings because it symbolizes another source of unpleasantness for the family.

Usually a family member must look backward in order to go forward. Grasping the meaning of what is currently happening in the family implies a fuller review and understanding, again of those past events that may have caused the loss. As family members review the past and express their feelings about the loss in a nonjudgmental context, and as they begin to understand the implications of the loss to family life, they are making progress toward adaptation and grief resolution. Adjustment to the loss involves change from the old ways of conducting family tasks to a different outlook for the future, modifications in family duties, and embracing new choices and opportunities.

Another difference in intervention approaches from those described in Chapter 6 is the helping "style" of health care professionals. They can often facilitate change by sharing their own feelings in uncertain situations and engaging in relevant and personal disclosure. When attending to other family concerns during the in-hospital treatment and outpatient rehabilitation phases, and when sharing of illness/disability-related information, including the identification of support resources, the grieving process that accompanies many of the family's unmet needs may be eventually resolved through the encouragement and willingness of the health care provider to reveal, when appropriate and helpful, personal feelings over what has happened to the family. This is not an easy task, but appropriate disclosure can provide valuable assistance during the family's grieving periods. Kane (1990), however, believes that effective helping with grief includes "maintaining a presence with the griever rather than solving the griever's problems ... not by attempting to remove the griever's pain, but instead, by allowing the griever to feel the pain of the loss" (p. 221). Walker and Pomeroy (1996) point out that caregivers who are grieving rather than depressed need support, using the full range of their emotions toward the care recipient without the expectation that they will reach a stage of acceptance in some orderly predictable fashion. When providing support, health care providers must be aware of their own empathy fatigue. Continued exposure to family members experiencing the grief associated with life-threatening illnesses and disabilities can promote burnout (Stebnicki, 2000).

When a family member, moreover, is experiencing the emotion of grief as a reaction to a serious loss, he/she will need to be motivated to break from the reaction in order to get on with grieving as coping (Attig, 1996). To break this hold may necessitate the realization that one is not a victim or helpless, and that there are choices. The choice to struggle against the attractions of grief can be a beginning step. Coming to terms with "letting go" can be a difficult task, but this resolve can introduce new experiences and patterns of life despite the real losses (Attig, 1996).

When planning family grief management approaches, McGoldrick (1991) reports several goals:

1. A shared acknowledgement that losses have occurred, implying that family members learn about the circumstances of the loss and face their own and each other's reactions to it.
2. Putting the loss into context, which may mean a review of family history, its culture, and the perspectives of different family members. When this knowledge is shared, it may help the family to integrate the loss experience into their lives by promoting a sense of familial, cultural, and human continuity. Family members can regain a sense of themselves as moving in time from the past, through the present, and into the future.
3. Reorganizing the family system, which may "entail a shift in caretaking roles or re-organizational and leadership functions, a reorientation of the social network . . . " (p. 55).
4. Redefining commitments and life priorities—these efforts may demand redirecting some relationships and focusing more clearly on what family members want to do in life and on how they wish to relate to others.

To assist the family to achieve these goals requires specialized skills and perspectives. The skills include the ability to access, create, and develop support mechanisms that inspire hope based on reality, but not limited to it (Quell, 2001). While reality can be a "common ground" for the family and the health care team, it can also be perceived differently. To the family, it can be overwhelming because they are engaged in a very subjective life experience compared with the objective frame of reference of the health care team. Occasionally, the reality demands for the caregiver may be in excess of current or future resources. This can create a desperate situation.

During the family visits, the health care provider assumes the role of a listener and a facilitator for the expression of feelings, and begins to comprehend and appreciate family dynamics. Active listening can help the family because it communicates an acceptance of the family and invites the family members to share their worries and anxieties. Active listening also promotes the opportunity for family members to express themselves, namely, to express feelings and complaints without being judged. A response such as "this is normal" is frequently the most reassuring information for the family. This is when support groups can help normalize the process and create a roadmap and benchmark for families.

Such professional roles, e.g., listener, and facilitator, are similar to other family meetings when attention to family grieving issues is not the primary focus of intervention. Another role, however, is providing information that is directed more on the losses associated with the chronic illness or severe disability. Although the loss may temporarily become the most striking feature of family life, the remaining resource opportunities should be emphasized. These resources are often the established family strengths or environmental supports readily available to family members. Providing information may frequently mean reinforcing health care knowledge, suggesting new expectations for the family members, or reviving expectations for each other that might have been lost at the onset of the medical event. When reflecting upon his work with the parents of a traumatically injured adolescent who died, Jacobs (1997) stated:

> When families are focused on proving the rehab experts wrong, it leads to an antagonistic and counterproductive relationship with the treatment team. It was my job to carve out the arenas of common perception from which we could all work together (p. 449).

During the family visits, and re-emphasizing the importance of reviewing past events, it also may necessary for family members to verbalize their feelings and then eventually make sense out of the loss. The family must ask the unanswerable "whys" over and over again before adjustment to the loss can begin to take place. Piece by piece, the links with the past are reexamined, grieved, given up, and partially replaced with the hope that what is lost may be compensated for or even replaced by another source of personal or family satisfaction. While it may be important for families to ask "why?" it may be more important for all involved to ask and understand "why not?"

While a timetable for loss and grief resolution cannot always be set (Kane, 1990), and the reactive experience among family members can be quite variable, a key consideration is to help the family cope in a constructive way and for family members to avoid making the situation worse by poor decisions, neglect, and maladaptive behaviors. What can contribute to this avoidance is for the health care provider to realize that there does not have to be immediate family rebuilding but rather family stabilization so the rebuilding process can begin when appropriate. Loss and bereavement is both a healing and rebuilding process.

Toward the conclusion of the family meetings, a plan of action could be developed that may take many forms. It can provide support, reassurance, role models, information to help the family members move through the grief process and/or utilize situational supports and resources. Having a variety of well-integrated resources available to a family encourages grief resolution. Pastoral care, neighborhood crisis clinics, and friends can provide valuable assistance during the bereavement period. Identifying with others through support groups often helps toward both acceptance of the loss and acknowledgement that changes should be made in family life. Contact with the local chapters of disability organizations and other resources can be helpful. While participation in these organizations and support groups is not a panacea for all of the issues and problems faced by a family, it provides the opportunity to learn from others who are in a similar situation and can provide another dimension for social interaction.

By supporting the learning of new information and skills while attending to each other's needs and expressing feelings, the family can begin the process of rebuilding, refocusing, and rejuvenating. This perspective is based upon the awareness that surviving and living beyond the event of a chronic illness or disability is hard work and that family members may not be able to progress at the same pace to reach their individual or common goals. Throughout the intervention, however, the family assumes the responsibility for any needed change.

With the bereaved family there may be a terminating phase, but the members usually want the opportunity for periodic dialogue with the initial health care professional during the time that characterizes adjustment to a medical situation. They may want someone they can turn to when the painful reality of the loss occasionally becomes overwhelming. Consequently, contact with the family is important until it is mutually perceived that the family is coping successfully and does not need or desire further involvement with the health care professional. This is where self-help groups play a significant role because they are often more understanding and readily available to the person with disability and his or her family.

CONCLUSION

A family loss related to a chronic illness/disability experience is a powerful, encompassing, and dynamic process. In order for family members to cope effectively they often need skillful and relevant intervention. This intervention must relate to the complexity of coping with the illness or injury (Stoler & Hill, 1998). Families need someone who can be there to listen, be a role model, offer reassurance, provide perspective, and validate their feelings. Intervention can take many forms but it is always guided by the conviction that underlying all approaches is the willingness to share another's loss as well as their hopes and dreams. Such sharing is frequently the beginning of a resolution of the family loss and recognition that life is livable even though it will never be exactly the same. The power of a hopeful perspective is that it creates a vision for the future, clarifies the present, and contains the past. As one spouse poignantly stated, "Don't ever take away our hope for recovery" (Mulder, 1998).

An intervention goal is to keep the family intact and to help members realize tht "life can be worth living" during and after the experience. Rolland (1994) states:

> A serious health crisis can awaken family members to opportunities for more satisfying, fulfilling relationships with each other. Hence any useful clinical model should emphasize the possibilities for growth, not just the liabilities and risks (p. 10).

In looking toward the future and transcending grief, Davidhizar (1997) emphasizes that people with disabilities do not have to remain at the grief stage. Rather, "they can learn to accept their disabilities and adapt to symptoms while maintaining normalcy in their lives. Although their sources of satisfaction may change, their life satisfaction can be maintained" (p. 35). Such a statement places the trauma and loss in a context, focuses on the future life to live, and it is not limited by the life that was lost.

GERALDINE: A DAUGHTER'S JOURNEY

This personal statement is the reflection of a mother faced with the illness and death of her eldest child at a most difficult point in time. Her child was also a young mother with a child and so much to live for. It is an account of the personal nature of loss and how family members have their own unique way to manage their grief. The mother's brief story also illustrates how courage tempered the impact of loss, and enabled her to maintain a positive quality of life while dealing with the reality of sorrow.

> On an early morning in February my daughter, Geraldine, discovered a lump in her breast. It was diagnosed as malignant and she then went through six

weeks of radiation after a lumpectomy. My daughter and son-in-law were very optimistic. After all, my daughter had a very strong will. She seemed to get what she wanted—queen of the prom, lead in the college play, dean's list in college, and what she considered the most desirable catch of all, marrying her husband, a young college professor. She was also certain most of the time that she could, in her own way, lick the cancer.

Seven months after detecting the lump in her breast, she discovered another lump in a lymph node in the left side of her neck, which was identified as cancerous. They were right in the midst of moving to a large university campus, and had decisions to make, namely, should they leave the clinic and their doctors and go immediately on chemo and radiation. After much consultation and deliberation her records were sent to their new home, and they were told to sit tight, though right after the move my daughter had an ovariectomy to slow down hormones. Through all of this, and certainly during the progression of the disease, I cried a lot, went out and worked, and felt a little angry, bitter, and jealous of other mothers who had their daughters. Prayer kept me going, and I kept thinking positively about what I would do to help her get better. I never gave up till the very last minute.

A few weeks after the operation my daughter and son-in-law came to New York and consulted more cancer specialists. But they both were extremely worried and realized that chemotherapy and radiation were devastating and felt it was the last thing. My daughter's husband seemed to cope by reading everything on cancer he could find, and his wife joined him in this reading. After returning to her son and husband in the Midwest, and a few weeks before December of that year, Geraldine started chemotherapy, was feeling better healthwise, and was glad something was being done. But the lump in her neck did not change though she tolerated the chemotherapy well, and after one week in the hospital she was put on an outpatient basis.

In December my daughter developed pneumonia and was hospitalized. My other daughter came to stay with her, but by the middle of the month she became very weak and dizzy and returned to New York. Her husband also obtained Laetrile, learned how to inject it, and when Geraldine came to New York, I had to do it. It was very difficult to plunge a needle into her buttock, but she insisted and felt sure it would help. Her husband "discovered" other cures, such as cloves, every vitamin imaginable, and eating only natural foods processed at home. He also spent nights reading in the medical library and became so knowledgeable that he could tell the doctors about new treatments and ideas on cancer.

After arriving in New York, Geraldine got progressively worse and became so weak we had to feed her. But every night she seemed a little better and then we would bathe her and we believed she was getting used to the Laetrile. She felt dizzy and went to the hospital the day after Christmas. A brain tumor was diagnosed. With radiation and cortisone she began to feel less dizzy and returned in early January to her home in the Midwest, though she needed a wheelchair to get around. Geraldine knew her husband and son needed her and often said her husband was keeping her alive. She also meditated and wished the cancer out of her body, prayed fervently, and did everything the doctors told her to do. At times she seemed very depressed, sad, and lonely, but said that she was not afraid. I know she seriously thought of suicide and asked me to forgive her if she did it. But she felt that, in some way, it would hurt her son.

In February she got pneumonia, followed by a urinary tract infection and strep throat. She was very sick and spent six weeks in the hospital. We all went to be with her, but Geraldine became very despondent and expressed the wish to die at home. She spoke of dying, which I listened to but tried to point out that she had youth, good genes, and desire to live on her side. I realized that she was not really in pain, but the mental anguish was terrible. That is the part that hurts me the most. I knew it was with Geraldine and her husband night and day. All the hopes and despair. Mental suffering is worse than physical.

Geraldine tried hypnosis, psychiatry, the charismatic movement, and put a lot of faith in a relic of Mother Seton. She really had a very strong will to live, but I think she knew that she would not. She was sad at leaving her son and since she knew her husband would be famous someday, she wanted very much to help him to achieve greatness. She also worried about who would take care of us when we were old.

Three months later there really was no change. She became extremely weak but remained lucid. On a weekend in May, she went to bed and the next day fell into a coma. We took her to the hospital and after five days in the coma, Geraldine died.

After many years, I still miss her dreadfully. I cry at very odd moments and am reminded of her a couple of times a day. Geraldine and I were very close and we so enjoyed our visits with each other. At first I had her pictures all around the house, but very soon I think I will put the one on my dresser away. It hurts too much to look at it, and I know I will never be the same. I was always a very happy person and felt that life was great. Now I think life can be cruel, and not for myself only since there is war, disease, and corruption, and I wonder what's it all about. Everyone has problems and troubles, but when Geraldine died, a part of me died—it could be my lust for life. People say time heals. But it is always there and pops up many times a day when I'm least expecting it. I just try to get over it and know life keeps going on and I cannot inflict my feelings on others. I have fared pretty well, and I am fortunate to have my husband and two other children who love me very much and I love them. I thank God for that.

DISCUSSION QUESTIONS

1. Considering the discussion of loss in this chapter, how did the mother and husband deal with the terminal illness of Geraldine?
2. What was the frame of reference that Geraldine and her mother had and discuss how it was an asset during the treatment process?
3. Why was Geraldine's family able to rally in a time of crisis?

SET 11: IS THE PERSON WITH AN ILLNESS OR DISABILITY MORE IMPORTANT THAN THE FAMILY?

PERSPECTIVE

The occurrence of a severe disability often focuses all of the family's emotional resources on the person who has sustained the disability. Often this focusing is essential to contain the fallout from the injury as well as to stabilize the total family system. However, in order for families to realign their goals and to establish a different balance in their lives while managing the impact of the loss, they must make a transition that considers the individual needs of family members, the total needs of the family, and the emerging, changing needs of the family member living with altered physical or emotional resources.

EXPLORATION

1. In coping with the demands of an illness or disability in your family, how did or would you allocate emotional resources? Why?
2. Is it ever possible to regain balance in the family following a major trauma? How is it done?
3. How long is a long time?

REFERENCES

Attig. T. (1996). *How we grieve.* New York: Oxford University Press.

Bader, J. L., & Robbins, R. (2001). Good grief! Helping families cope. *Volta Voices, 8*(4), 28–29.

Bowlby, J. (1980). *Attachment and loss: Loss, sadness and depression,* Vol 3. New York: Basic Books.

Brown, J.C. (1990). Loss and grief: An overview and guided imagery intervention model. *Journal of Mental Health Counseling, 12*(4), 434–445.

Bugen, L. A. (1977). Human grief: A model for prediction and intervention. *American Journal of Orthopsychiatry, 47,* 196–206.

Davidhizar, R. (1997). Disability does not have to be the grief that never ends: Helping patients adjust. *Rehabilitation Nursing, 22*(1), 32–35.

Davis, B. H. (1987). Disability and grief. *The Journal of Contemporary Social Work,* June, 352–358.

Doka, K. J. (1995). *Children mourning, mourning children.* Washington, DC: Hospice Foundation of America.

Fell, M. (1994). Helping older children grieve: A group therapy approach. *Health Visitor, 67*(3), 92–94.

Garner, J. (1997). Dementia: An intimate death. *British Journal of Medical Psychology, 70*(2), 177–184.

Jacobs, B. J. (1997). In sickness and health: Seeing and believing. *Families, Systems, & Health, 15*(4), 447–457.

Kane, B. (1990). Grief and the adaptation to loss. *Rehabilitation Education, 4,* 213–224.

Kapust, L. R., & Weintraub, S. (1984). Living with a family member suffering from Alzheimer's disease. In H. D. Roback (Ed.), *Helping patients and their families cope with medical problems.* San Francisco: Jossey-Bass.

Livneh, H., & Antonak, R. F. (1997). *Psychosocial adaptation to chronic illness and disability.* Gaithersburg, MD: Aspen.

Lyons, R. F., & Sullivan, M. (1998). Curbing loss in illness and disability: A relationship perspective. In J. H. Harvey (Ed.), *Perspectives on loss: A sourcebook.* New York: Brunner/Mazel.

Matz, M. (1978). Helping families cope with grief. In S. Eisenberg & L. Patterson (Eds.), *Helping clients with special concerns.* Chicago: Rand McNally.

McGoldrick, M. (1991). Echoes from the past: Helping families mourn their losses. In F. Walsh & M. McGoldrick (Eds.), *Living beyond loss: Death in the family.* New York: Norton.

McGoldrick, M., Hines, P. M., Garcia-Preto, N., Almeida, R., Rosen, E., & Lee, E. (1991). Mourning in different cultures. In F. Walsh & M. McGoldrick (Eds.), *Living beyond loss: Death in the family.* New York: Norton.

Miller, T.W., Houston, L., & Goodman, R. (1994). Clinical issues in psychosocial rehabilitation for spouses with physical disabilities. *Journal of Developmental and Physical Disabilities, 6*(1), 50.

Mulder, P. (1998). Proceeding 17, TBI Challenge Symposium, December 2, 9. Brain Injury Association, Alexandria, VA.

Osterweis, M., Solomon, F., & Green, M. (Eds.) (1984). *Bereavement: Reactions, consequences, and care.* Washington, DC: National Academy Press.

Parkes, C. M. (1975). Determinants of outcome following bereavement. *Omega, 6,* 303–323.

Pollock, G. H. (1961). Mourning and adaptation. *International Journal of Psychoanalysis, 42,* 341–361.

Power, P. W., & Dell Orto, A. E. (2003). *The resilient family.* Notre Dame, IN: Sorin Books.

Quell, B. (2001). Living well: Disability, grief, and loss. *PN/Paraplegia News, 55*(8), 27.

Rolland, J. S. (1994). *Families, illness and disability: An integrative treatment model.* New York: Basic Books.

Romanoff, B. D. (1993). When a child dies: Special considerations for providing mental health counseling for bereaved parents. *Journal of Mental Health Counseling, 15*(4), 384–393.

Stebnicki, M. A. (2000). Stress and grief reactions among rehabilitation professionals: Dealing effectively with empathy fatigue. *Journal of Rehabilitation, 66*(1), 23–29.

Stoler, D. R., & Hill, B. A. (1998). *Coping with mild traumatic brain injury.* Garden City, NY: Avery Publishing Group.

Stroebe, M., Gergen, M., Gergen, K., & Stroebe, W. (1992). Broken hearts or broken bonds: Love and death in historical perspective. *American Psychologist, 47*(10), 1205–1212.

Walker, R. J., & Pomeroy, E. C. (1996). Depression or grief? The experience of caregivers of people with dementia. *Health and Social Work, 21*(4), 247–254.

Walsh, F., & McGoldrick, M. (1991). *Living beyond loss: Death in the family.* New York: Norton.

Weisman, A. (1973). Coping with untimely death. *Psychiatry, 36*, 366–378.

Whiston, S. C. (2000). *Principles and applications of assessment in counseling.* Belmont, CA: Wadsworth/Thomson.

Worden, W. (1991). *Grief counseling and grief therapy* (2nd ed.) New York: Springer.

Wright, H., & Oliver, G. (1993). *Kids have feelings too.* Chicago: Victor Books

Zemzars, L. S. (1984). Adjustment to health loss: Implications for psychosocial treatment. In S. E. Milligan (Ed.), *Community health care for chronic physical illness.* Cleveland, OH: Case Western Reserve University.

Reflections and Considerations

INTRODUCTION

Prior chapters have presented the impact of illness and disability on the family from a life and living perspective. This perspective attempts to put the past in a functional context, maximizes the opportunities of present, and anticipates a future enhanced by optimism, tempered by reality, and enriched with hope. This final chapter will 1) reflect upon some of the issues and complications related to the family's illness and disability experience, 2) discuss some possible myths that may be part of a person's or family's frame of reference, 3) explore selected research topics that may influence future coping and adaptation, and 4) identify the specific issues of expectations, compassion, hope, and spirituality which are important dimensions when assisting families experiencing severe illness and disability.

REFLECTIONS

For those persons and families living the illness and disability experience, the past is unalterable, but the future can be somewhat controlled, even though it is very uncertain and unpredictable. When the impact and consequences of loss and change are most prominent in a family's life, there is always the temptation to replay the past and rethink the causal events, while hoping for a different or more palatable outcome (e.g., if I only I had made them wear a seatbelt they would not be disabled; if I had encouraged my wife to stop smoking she would not have lung cancer: if I had not told her that she must take the job in the World Trade Center, rather than going to school as she wanted to,

---

*Some of the material in this chapter is updated and modified from Dell Orto & Power, 2000 and Power, Dell Orto, & Gibbons, 1988. Reprinted with permission.

she would be alive today). Decisions were made and the consequences are permanent and have major implications for all involved.

When individuals and families experience and bear witness to the causes and consequences of many illnesses and disabilities, there is the drive and commitment to make sure that it does not happen again. In fact, having an illness or disability does not guarantee that a person will not have another that could be better or worse. For example, the possibility of another illness or disability is actually increased the longer we live and the more exposure we have, e.g., being on the highway, on vacation, or at work includes risk for life altering experiences.

Similarly, in some cases when successful rehabilitation interventions have increased independence and expanded life domains, there is an increased vulnerability to the very risks families are attempting to master and control. Consider the reaction of a family awarded two million dollars in a personal injury case for their traumatically injured 17-year-old daughter. They bought her a sports car and, as a result, she was in a car accident because she was speeding and drinking. She became a quadriplegic and her brother was killed. At this point, her mother stated that their situation went from bad to worse—which she never could have imagined. The money promised a lot of hope, but delivered a great deal of pain. She added that they all would have been better off without it.

It is at this point that families are confused, angry, and vulnerable. The issue is not only who can be blamed or can pay, but also what can be done to validate the person living with the consequences and make the life care process more reasonable. The problem is that no amount of money can regain what was lost, undo the pain and sorrow, and guarantee that life will be easier on all fronts. While money can certainly relieve the financial burden and provide the resources needed to enhance quality of life, it can also cause additional unanticipated problems and difficulties.

Large cash settlements have distorted the issues and created a caste system. Some families must ask: "Why should someone else with a traumatic injury similar to my child's be awarded a multimillion dollar settlement and get the best of care while my child lives in squalor with a broken wheelchair and without personal care attendants just because he was injured by a person without insurance or even resources?" This is one of the many challenges facing health care and rehabilitation today. A system must be developed that is based upon human value, respect for life, and family stabilization that includes more than are excluded. No cost is too great if it is helping those who have too little. Any cost is too great if helps those who do not need it at the expense of those who do.

This is an ongoing complexity of life: there are no guarantees, only opportunities, choices, and consequences. We cannot prevent the inevitable, but we must try to provide meaningful intervention, nonjudgmental support, and consistent caring. However, it is critical that interventions be based on a realistic perspective of the human condition as it is and as it will become. People are in a constant state of growth and deterioration. We cannot be immunized from the human experience even if we or others are focused on this as a noble goal.

Callahan in his book, *False Hopes: Overcoming the Obstacles to a Sustainable, Affordable Medicine* (1999), makes some important points that have a direct bearing on how people and families respond to health and its deterioration:

> By its tacit implication that in the quest for health lies, perhaps, the secret of the meaning of life, modern medicine has misled people into thinking that the ills of the flesh, and mortality itself, are not to be understood and integrated into a balanced view of life but simply to be fought and resisted. It is as if the medical struggle against illness, aging and death is itself the source of (or at least a source of) human meaning. I refer not only to the almost religious devotion some have to improving their health and their bodies so that health itself becomes the goal of life, but also the idea that, in an other-wise meaningless world, the effort to relieve suffering becomes a source of meaning.

Many families find themselves in very complicated and demanding situations in which their medical condition cannot be improved or improvement could be made but the needed resources are not available or accessible. Loss and change are undeniable dimensions and forces of the human experience. Consequently, every effort should be made to help the person and family live their lives with human dignity and values that appreciate life, accept mortality, recognize vulnerability, promote hope, and demonstrate caring. Some of the most poignant statements a family can make are "we should have," "if only," "why us?" Rarely do people say, "why not?"

COMPLICATIONS

Families may also find themselves in situations where the solution to the presenting problem creates more problems than were expected or anticipated. The emotionality and complexity of the issues related to cardiopulmonary resuscitation, for example, and the burden placed on families who are hoping for full recoveries while faced with losses are discussed by Phipps (1998):

> Because families view rehabilitation, at least initially, with a hopefulness for the patient's full recovery, initiating discussions of this topic early on in the rehabilitation process may be experiences as too emotionally burdensome to yield informed decisions and may be viewed as counterproductive to establishing trust and rapport. Some families appear to welcome talk about their own concerns, while others do not want to or are unable to grapple with the topic. Families who ultimately choose against resuscitation for their family member may have shifted in their hopefulness about the patient's recovery; may have lived with a patient with a chronic debilitating illness and believe that should the patient arrest, resuscitation may not be in the patient's best interest or possibly not in theirs (p. 97).

An alternative perspective on complications and unanticipated problems is the great appreciation families have for those heroic efforts which have kept their loved ones alive and have given them the chance to continue life but at a different level. As a wife stated:

> One day I have a husband who is the strength of the family, who makes everyone proud, and the next, I have this person who scares everyone with his temper and who thinks everything is fine when it's a sorry mess. But life is getting better. The two of us get along. Sometimes I even like the fact that my husband is around all the time. He can be good company . . . I guess we'll be a good old twosome until the day we die . . . Life is hard. I'm a survivor (Dell Orto & Power, 2000).

In both of these examples, the common element is that the families are going to have to live with the consequences of their unique life experience. The challenge for society and health care is to provide the support, encouragement, and role models needed to keep illness and disability in perspective so that it does not become a ravaging force that destroys the family that is trying to survive against great odds.

Assisting families to cope with illness and disability is often a lifelong process. It demands creative efforts on the part of the health care and rehabilitation teams, as well as the commitment and investment of team members who are sensitive to and aware of the needs of the person and the family living an experience of ongoing change, loss, and perhaps even potential gains.

SELECTED MYTHS

A challenge is to approach health care, treatment, and rehabilitation from an optimistic as well as realistic perspective. This is not an easy task since there are many myths which can influence family expectations during the treatment and rehabilitation process. Some of these myths are described below.

MYTH 1: ILLNESS AND DISABILITY CAN BE PREVENTED OR CURED

While it is a noble goal to reduce all of the precipitating and causal factors related to the incidence of illness and disability, no amount of education or prevention will eradicate all the variables, conditions, and situations that cause illness and disability such as drunk driving, drug-related violence, war, crime, guns, alcohol, drugs, poor diet, genetics, poverty, accidents, terrorism, sports injuries, abuse, toxic environments, work injuries, cars, bicycles, or just the reality of the life and living process. And sometimes, even though there are helpful guidelines (e.g., seatbelt use, exercise, bicycle helmets, smoking cessation), there are many people who continue to engage in behaviors that place their health or that of their family a risk. An irony is that cars do hit some joggers in pursuit of wellness. Some have minor injuries, while others are severely injured or killed.

MYTH 2: RESTORATION IS MORE IMPORTANT THAN REALISTIC ACCEPTANCE

While significant gains have been made in illness and disability prevention, treatment, and rehabilitation, there are some voids which cannot be filled but which must be crossed, sometimes with the body, other times by the spirit. This may be an ultimate challenge for persons and families faced with the choice between retrieving who they were and accepting who they are now and who they are becoming.

Illness and disability will always be with us. So will hope, creativity, cure, restoration, and resilience. Approaching illness, disability, and aging in a holistic, caring, creative, and visionary way has the potential to enrich and enhance the quality of life of the person living with unique life circumstances as well as that of the family.

MYTH 3: SOMEONE MUST PAY

For many families enduring the journey of treatment and rehabilitation, the idea that "someone must pay" can be a potential emotional and financial trap. Emotionally, a family may feel they have been wronged—

and often justifiably so. For example, a family may feel a drunk driver, whose actions placed a child in a coma management program, has wronged them. But what if this person is uninsured, a repeat offender, or has no resources? Who becomes the object of attention? Is it the media who promote alcohol use and abuse or the manufacturers who portray reckless driving in their ads? Is it the employer who unjustly fires a person who then becomes angry and shoots a coworker resulting in a severe injury? What about the elderly driver whose poor skills and judgment cause a car accident and a subsequent injury or death of a child?

A great amount of emotional and physical of energy can be expended in focusing on the cause and circumstances related to the losses,illness, and disability. When all is said and done, the family may or may not be responsible for the problem, but they have the opportunity to be responsible for the solution.

MYTH 4: THE FAMILY AND THE INDIVIDUAL WILL ALWAYS APPRECIATE MEDICAL INTERVENTION

Another myth that creates stress for families is the expectation that all medical intervention is helpful and will be beneficial. When discussing catastrophic illness and disability, families and health care professionals must be able to discuss some very controversial, emotional, and difficult issues related to the cost, benefit, and effort related to intervention and outcome. For example, while some families are very happy that their family member's life was saved, even though there are severe limitations, other families may not be as pleased. This can occur as the long-term reality of the situation is comprehended and the future is more dismal than uplifting.

This point is well-illustrated by the pain expressed by a mother who encouraged the heroic efforts made by the medical team that saved her son's life after an industrial accident, but a year after, when he was not making progress and his quality of life was deteriorating she stated, "They just prevented him from dying." Now, from her perspective, both he and his family are relegated to an emotional and physical prison. Apart from the financial costs and physical and emotional toll, the outcome has been individual stress and familial chaos.

MYTH 5: UNQUESTIONING FAITH IN THE HEALTH CARE TEAM AND SYSTEM

In some situations the needs of the family are secondary to the goals, interests, and resources of the people and systems involved in the care of a family member. Also, there are the inherent problems in the health care system that can make problems worse.

This is often an alien concept for families who have looked toward these resources and systems from an overly optimistic frame of reference. Families must often advocate for themselves if they cannot align themselves with people and systems that can provide relevant and meaningful support.

While most health care professionals do their very best to provide the best of care for their patients, there are some situations, as reflected in the following comments, that are painful and do not have clear answers or easy resolutions:

- A veteran was asked, "Who took your leg off? A shoemaker?"
- A mother stated "I wish we had insisted on a mastectomy, rather than a lumpectomy. Then maybe she would still be alive."
- The doctor told us there would be no problems and never mentioned the possibility of death. We would never have had the corrective surgery.
- The nurses and doctors asked me why would I ever have another child after the birth of two severely disabled children.
- The doctor said to us, "If you had had the child in our hospital she would not have spina bifida."

MYTH 6: TECHNOLOGY WILL PROVIDE ALL THE ANSWERS

Without doubt, technology has enhanced the lives of people with illness and disability and has increased the options and opportunities in the life, learning, and working domains. However, for some families existing technology may not be relevant to the needs of their family members or may not be accessible. This creates a unique set of stressors for the person and family faced with conditions and situations that are not resolved by technology.

MYTH 7: MY FAMILY WILL ALWAYS BE THERE FOR ME BECAUSE I WAS THERE FOR THEM

Some families have expended a great amount of energy on caregiving for other family members. A point of great stress occurs when they are in need and the family or its members are not there for them. As one person said, "I gave up a career and a family for you and now you do not have time for me? What a surprise and a major disappointment!" On the other hand there may be family members who have been outside of the family life and who emerge as positive forces in times of need. An example of this is a relative who was shunned by the family due to his life-style but who offered a kidney to a relative. This changed the family dynamic for the better.

MYTH 8: IF WE ARE GOOD TO OTHERS AND EVEN PROVIDE FINANCIAL ASSISTANCE, CAREGIVING, AND RESPITE CARE, THEY WILL BE GOOD TO US OR RESPOND IN KIND

While this may occur, there are some situations where no matter what is done for others, family included, their response to the needs of those who have been responsive to them may be far less than ideal. Often this is the basis for many family conflicts and part of intergeneration issues and cutoffs. It is within this life and living perspective that many of the issues related to illness and disability, loss and change, treatment and rehabilitation, are cast in a different light.

RESEARCH

While there is great value in ongoing family-relevant research, the emerging information must be assessed and considered in the context of how it impacts families and their abilities to process, integrate, and benefit from the data and policy generated. This point was emphasized in a report from the Agency for Health Care Policy and Research (1998):

> In addition to outcomes of changed patient functionality, there should be outcomes of changed family functionality. Since much of case management communication is directed toward helping family members learn what to expect and where to obtain services, relevant outcomes would include family use of community and rehabilitation services and indicators of family assert-iveness about care expectations (p. 8).

In the discussion of challenges in family health intervention research, Kazak (2002) stated:

> The argument has been made that the extraordinary stress associated with chronic illness heightens vulnerability to psychological difficulties and even psychiatric diagnosis. While there is increased vulnerability, the generally adaptive functioning of most patients translates into adaptive coping for many

(if not most), episodic difficulties for some, and may provoke or coexist with more serious psychosocial or psychiatric problems for a minority. One of the major challenges to researchers in this field is to identify whether intervention will be directed towards the generally well-coping majority, the selected group of families with distressing and probably episodic problems, or the subset that is likely to have multiple, ongoing, and potentially disabling psychological difficulties (p. 54).

Consequently, family-focused research should address what families will need from different perspectives (Weihs, Fisher, & Baird, 2002). Kazak (2002) provides the following recommendations:

1. Use information of family risk and protective factors to design selective interventions that target the patients and families who lack resilience for disease management.
2. Emphasize family assessment prior to intervention to determine for which kinds of families the intervention worked and for which it did not.
3. Explore the use of noncategorical disease intervention programs.
4. Consider patient gender and family ethnicity as core concepts in designing family-focused interventions (p. 51).

These recommendations have a proactive dimension and sensitivity to the unique life and cultural experiences of families. Without these perspectives it is often presumptuous to decide what families are willing and capable of doing for themselves and for each other.

Given the demands faced by some families and individuals who may feel depersonalized and their quality of life diminished by today's health care system, Halstead (2001) stated:

> In today's high-tech impersonal health care system the use of scientific methods to show that humanistic treatments are effective may represent a new frontier and an opportunity for rehabilitation research (p. 149).

EXPECTATIONS

To expect the family to provide support to a member in need implies that the health care and rehabilitation team, as well as policy makers, are very aware of the rigors of treatment, rehabilitation, and recovery, and their impact on the family. They should appreciate, comprehend, and value the costs and rewards of adjusting to illness and disability, as well as the importance of assisting the family to stabilize, recover, and grow. To facilitate the process of learning, coping, and surviving, the family needs timely and relevant interventions, appropriate skills, and accessible support. When these needs are met, the family's reactions to and decisions about themselves and the person with an illness or disability can be made from a position of strength rather than from desperation and frustration.

Often the individual and family problems are related not only to the illness and/or disability concerns, but also consequent to the resources and supports. This does not mean that in all situations more resources and supports will result in more positive outcomes. It does imply that in many situations family problems can be addressed and responded to in an active and helpful way. Unfortunately, some of the basic needs of families are being considered as luxuries in the current health care environment when, in fact, they are essential and often critical. This is most alarming given the recent RAND report published in *The New England Journal of Medicine* in June 2003, and referenced in *The New York Times,* on July 2, 2003:

> A study published last week in the *New England Journal of Medicine* found that participants whose medical records were analyzed had failed to get the recommended treatment for their illnesses almost half the time (p. A22).

Marginalization of patients and minimization of services by health care providers are often part of the driving force behind the family's outrage, disappointment, and distress. This energy may be redirected to focus on empowerment, advocacy, and other consumer movements that have set a course to meet the needs of families living with illness and disability experiences in spite of organizational obstacles, policy limitations, and competing interests for scarce and dwindling resources.

Occasionally, there is a rational framework which facilitates the acceptance of this reality, e.g., that older persons have reached retirement age, have lived fulfilling lives, fulfilled their responsibilities, and had their physical, emotional, and cognitive abilities modified by the normal, or abnormal, conditions of aging. This point in life for some, however, also has its unique variations. Some elders are pleased with their lives, others are frustrated and or disappointed by what has, or has not, occurred. This is often intensified by the realization that options are confined and limited by the limited time individuals may have and the urgency to maximize what time and opportunities may be left for them.

The deterioration of an elderly person is a painful process, but it is more understandable than the randomness of illnesses and disabilities which assault children, adolescents, and adults at the most inopportune times of their lives. This is compounded by the fact that many illnesses and disabilities are a result of choices, actions, and behaviors which make accepting the irreversible consequences of accidents, lifestyle, trauma, and irrational violence difficult, at best, while raising a multitude of complex issues (Callahan, 1987; Phipps, 1998).

The situation becomes even more complicated when the solutions to the problems at hand do not meet, or even approximate, the hopes, aspirations, or expectations of the person or the family. It is at this point when families need the support and resources derived from compassion, hope, and spirituality.

COMPASSION

A powerful counterbalance to the stressors related to family illness and disability is active and responsive compassion. Blaylock (2000) reflected on compassion, the difficult situations families often face during treatment, and some of their needs:

> Patients and families are asked to endure debilitating treatments for the sake of a long-term goal, thrust into difficult caretaker roles, and called upon to cope with wrenching ethical dilemmas. In return they want compassion, respect, and information delivered in sensitive manner (p. 161).

During the health care and rehabilitation process it is important to note the importance and value of compassion as well as relationship-centered care by the health care team (Williams, Frankel, Campbell, & Deci, 2000).

In a discussion of compassion and caring, Halstead, 2001 stated:

> Rehabilitation of persons with catastrophic illness or injuries is a complex, labor-intensive interaction between patients and caregivers. Experiences of overwhelming loss and suffering evoke strong emotions that shape the behavior of both patients and staff during the rehabilitation process. In response to each patient's unique experience, compassion, caring, and other humanistic qualities of the effective caregiver help create a healing environment (p. 149).

HOPE

Illness, disability, and other major life changes transform and challenge the entire family system. This process has the power to confuse the present, distort the past, and compromise the future. It also creates familial stress and disappointment, as well as the conditions for healing and hope. Hope has emerged as an important consideration in the life and living process that is affected by illness and disability (Gottschalk, 1985; Nunn, 1996; Magaletta & Oliver, 1999; Scheier & Carver, 1992, 1998: Snyder, Irving, & Anderson, 1991). Hope is also a vital force in the families' journeys to move beyond what was and begin to understand and accept what is and what could be. The challenge can seem like transforming "millstones into stepping stones," which is not an easy task.

Many times families and individuals find themselves in situations where they are hopeless and/or hopeful and need responses that are relevant or useful at the present or in the future. A mother illustrated this point when she stated, "When my son was in the trauma unit it was not helpful to hear the long list of what he would never be able to do. We both needed some hope or something to move toward. I would never take that away from people even though what they would hope for may not happen."

The power and comfort of hope is reflected in a statement made by a friend of the author who was at the end of her life after a long experience with cancer. This very spirited 35-year-old woman, wife, and mother said, "I know I am dying, but as crazy as it sounds I still have hope. While I would like to live and hope for a miracle, at the same time I hope for the health, happiness, joy, and well-being of my family and friends. This gives me great comfort. While I am not that religious, I also hope that will be another dimension where I can enjoy the future of my family. This is my hope." This woman died two hours after making this statement, and we can only hope her wishes were met.

It is important that families be helped to recognize the difference between hope based on desperation and hope based on reality. For some families hope is what keeps them going and denial may be a means to keeping hope alive. Rather than forcing the family to rush beyond where they are ready to be, there is a need to appreciate why they are where they are and facilitate the support that enables them to stabilize their situation, energize their resources, and maximize their potential. This is where self-help organizations and support groups can helped develop functional perspectives for persons and families living in a twilight zone of confusion, pain, and overwhelming need. While the "storm" of illness and disability may not be avoided, the accessibility to "safe harbors" can make surviving possible.

SPIRITUALITY

The relationship of spirituality to disability and illness is appearing with growing frequency in the research literature (Kay & Raghaven, 2000).

Spirituality itself is the universal human desire for transcendence and connectedness (Carson, 1993). It spans the entire developmental life process, and includes participation in worship, prayer, and a sense of closeness to something greater than the self (Reed 1991; Koestenbaum, 1977).

McColl, Bickenback, Johnston, Nishihama, Schumaher, Smith, Smith, & Yealland (2000) concluded:

> Individuals with recently acquired disabilities were able to speak with candor and eloquence about changes to the spiritual self that had occurred in the wake of the onset of disability. Approximately half of the sample identified an appreciable loss or gain in faith at the time of their injury (p. 821).

For some, spirituality and religion are primary resources in understanding, comprehending, and negotiating the disability and illness experience. Kay and Raghavan (2002) stated that spirituality is a resource when dealing with critical and terminal illnesses, and that both patients and family members utilize it. In fact, "family members dealing with a critical illness report use of greater spiritual perspective" (Kay & Raghaven, 2002, p. 236). They need spiritual resources while caring for the sick person, and the individual with a disability or illness uses different spiritual activities to find purpose and meaning and a sense of hope for the future (Carroll, 1993; Young, 1993). Reflecting on his life threatening experience, Herbert (2003) also stated:

> One consequence of facing life-threatening or life-altering surgery is that it provides an opportunity to reflect on your life. For the first time, I began to think of my mortality and, in particular, my personal relationship with God (p. 125).

In effect, major life changes related to illness and disability may create new dimensions for the spirituality of the family.

CONCLUSION

A common goal most people have is to attain or maintain a reasonable quality of life for themselves, their family, or significant others. Often this is within the context of their past, present, or future reality. A major step in the process of life goal attainment is the realization that illness and disability are dynamic forces that will influence this process.

An illness or disability experience has great variability for those who are living the process. For some it is the greatest loss, for some it is just bearable. For others it is an opportunity for personal as well familial growth and enhancement. This may occur when the family is able to embrace the potential of what remains and not be consumed by the sorrow of what has been lost.

While more prominent for some more so than others, illness and disability are not the only challenges individuals and families must consider or respond to, but they are often the ones that will test many family's convictions, values, resources, and fortitude. The realities of change, loss, illness, disability, and aging can never be totally eliminated, but living with their consequences and implications certainly can be made more bearable.

CHRIS AND HIS MOTHER: HOPE AND HOME RUNS, NOT STRIKEOUTS

The following personal statement presents the often irrational life experiences that can test and strengthen the human mind, body, and spirit. A son and his mother share their journey, as well as the hopes and dreams that had to be let go as well as aspired to.

CHRIS'S PERSPECTIVE

Prior to my injury in July 1991, my family had endured its share of trials and tribulations. I guess you could say we were a typical middle-class family. At least we considered ourselves middle class. Actually we were on the low-income end of middle class, but we were happy. We never felt deprived of anything; even though we didn't have a lot of money for clothes or extras, we never went without. My two older brothers and I shared many wonderful times with our parents. Everyone was always very close: church every Sunday, dinners together, and always discussions on how things were going. My parents, to my knowledge, never missed a sporting event or school function. Everyone was treated fairly, given the same opportunities, and encouraged to grow and learn by experiencing new things. We were always given the freedom to choose our activities, but we were expected not to quit halfway through. If we started something, we were always expected to give it a fair chance before deciding not to continue with it. I guess that's where I developed much of my determination.

My father and mother shared the responsibilities of keeping the household going. When my father lost his job, he took over all the household chores and my mother continued to work full time. Dad was always the athletic type and he instilled in us the belief that hard work, determination, and self-confidence would not only help us athletically, but later in our lives as we began to go out into the world. Our friends were always welcome in our house. I'll never forget how my Dad would fix lunch every day for me and my best friend during our senior year. There aren't too many guys who would want to go home every day for lunch, but I always felt very comfortable with it.

Mom has always been the matriarch of the family. Being an optimist, she is able to see the good in everything. Although she's a petite woman, she has a quiet, gentle strength about her. I never tried to "pull one over on her," since she always had a way of finding things out. When one of us boys would do something we shouldn't have, Mom always found out. This still amazes me.

My oldest brother was always quiet and kind of shy. Acting as a role model for me and my other brother, he worked hard in school and pursued extracurricular activities. At the time of my injury he was out of school and living on his own. As the middle child, my other brother was more aggressive and outgoing. Striving for independence, he couldn't wait to be out on his own. As the youngest of the three boys, I was always on the go. I was very popular in school and gifted athletically. I had just graduated from high school and had secured a baseball scholarship at a nearby university. It had always been my dream to play professional ball. It seemed I had been preparing my *whole life* to play in the "big show." Little did I know that I was really preparing for the challenge of my life.

After graduating from high school I was carefree and looked forward to a great future. I was planning on attending Walsh University, where I had been awarded a baseball scholarship, where I would major in business. I could not wait to start college, become independent, and meet new people. New challenges and new opportunities occupied my thoughts.

The summer after my graduation was a time I remember vividly. Playing 80-odd games in six weeks and enjoying my new freedom with friends, I thought I had it all. I figured as long as I had baseball, friends, and family, I had everything I would ever need. What I did not figure on was losing baseball, being separated from friends, and becoming almost completely dependent on my family.

On July 29, 1991, a friend and I went to the mall to do some school shopping. Afterwards we decided to hang out at the local strip and see what was going on. We ran into two of our friends, Valerie and Bobby Joe.

The four of us talked and cruised around enjoying the cool summer night. Around 10:30 p.m. we decided to stop off at Taco Bell to go to the restroom and get some drinks. When we entered the Taco Bell I noticed nothing unusual so we proceeded to order. It was supposed to be a fun night out on the town and it probably would have ended that way had the conclusion of the night not found me lying in a coma, fighting for my life.

As we were leaving the restaurant I still hadn't noticed anything unusual. As I proceeded out the door a couple of steps behind my friends, I was struck in the face by a fist. Swinging around to see who had struck me, I was disoriented. As soon as I swung around, I felt a glass bottle shatter over my right temporal lobe. I immediately fell to the ground where I was kicked and beaten for what felt like an eternity, but was actually only a few minutes. Afterwards I slowly tried to regain consciousness. I was rushed to the hospital where I fell into a coma for a month.

Emerging from my coma was the greatest challenge of my life, a challenge I will never forget. It called for every resource I had if I were to breathe and walk again. It was like I was alone in a dense, thick fog groping for a familiar hand, yet unable to find anything concrete and strangely aware of a vast emptiness and solitude. This is a faint reflection of my coma. As I lay there, I experienced repeated flashes of light . . . my brain inevitably reacted. I wondered where the light came from! Had I really seen it or was it only a figment of my imagination? I convinced myself that the flash of light was real and, thus, my only hope of finding my way back home. From a great distance, I heard the distinct voices of my mother, father, and brothers, and Amy, the girl next door. Each time I heard their encouragement, I drew one step closer to the light. Although I felt like falling into despair, a word of love from God, my family, and my friends urged me forward. Without such love I would not have advanced even one step. Along with these words of love, I also heard the muffled voices of doctors and the high-pitched whispers of nurses as they wondered what they could do to help me. Eventually, they concluded that I would not make it. I was determined to prove them wrong.

Every day, I fought the coma with all of my might. Every day, I drew a little closer to the light. Finally, the day came when I opened my eyes and saw the heartbroken tears of the people I loved and longed to be with. Meanwhile, I could not move a single muscle in my body. I could not even talk. However, this did not bring my spirits down; somewhere deep within I knew that I had just answered the greatest challenge of all, the challenge of coming back from virtual death.

After awakening from my coma I slowly began to realize what had happened. I went from a fully functional young adult to practically a vegetable in a blink of an eye. I was left totally immobile, not able to talk and my world had seemed to crumble to dust. My family and friends were there to support me; if not for them I think I would have died.

During the ensuing weeks, the doctors and nurses gave me little hope for recovery, but through persistent pleading, my mother convinced the doctors to give me time before decisions were made to institutionalize me. My family and I vowed to meet this brain injury head on and give it our best. I slowly regained mobility and could see gradual improvements. The doctors also saw my progress and decided to send me to a rehabilitation hospital to continue therapy.

It was at the rehabilitation hospital that my attitude and commitment to recovery preceded all other thoughts. My family, friends, therapist, nurses, and doctors were my team and they were counting on me to bring them to victory. You see, it was the ninth inning, the game was tied, the bases were loaded, and I was at the plate facing a full count. It was the kind of situation I thrived on. It was do or die time. I could dig in, face the challenge, and try, or I could drop my bat, strike out, and die. The choice was mine. What did I do? Well, I stepped up to the box, dug my feet in, and my mind focused on the pitcher, or in this case the injury. I saw the ball coming; it was like a balloon. I stepped toward the ball, made a smooth swing, and then I heard a crack. The ball ricocheted off my bat like a bullet from a gun. I just stood there and watched it soar high and long; I knew in an instant it was gone. As I touched each base, a part of my recovery passed, and before I knew it, I was home, starting school, and enjoying life again.

Although my recovery is not yet complete, I play a game every day in my head, and with every hit, catch, and stolen base, a part of my recovery passes. My next home run could be the one that brings me full circle. The pursuit of this dream is encompassed by the determination and hope that one day I will make it back to my ball field. All I can do is try and pray that everything will turn out right, and if it does not, I will still go on because I know I gave it my best.

The road to recovery has been long and wearisome, but I have already put many miles behind me and I know I will emerge completely triumphant. This experience has taught me many valuable lessons. Above all, it has convinced me that the human will can overcome obstacles that many consider insurmountable. I have walked through the valley of the shadow of death and have come out, not unscathed but undaunted. I am among the few people who can say that they have experienced near-death and were able to live and talk about it. I consider myself lucky and remain grateful to all who have helped me recover from this disaster. My experience has indisputably helped make me the person I am today.

Although many things helped my family overcome this catastrophe, the most helpful was first and foremost our faith in God and belief that He would make everything all right. Second, was the overwhelming support we received from family and friends. How could we not make it with such kindness and compassion? Third, was becoming knowledgeable about brain injury. This seemed to make us feel more in control of the situation, instead of relying on doctors and nurses for details of what was happening. Throughout the injury, we kept a positive outlook on life, knowing that we would pull through. The family, as a whole, had a kind of inner strength, which told each member things would work out in the end. Finally, we came to accept the situation and the consequences it has brought. The past cannot be changed, but the present and future can.

Intervention was never offered to my family. I often wonder why, but I guess no one ever thought to ask what the family needed. Intervention that would have been helpful to my family includes:

- A team of doctors that would offer in-depth knowledge on the subject of head injury, or offer literature or reading material in lay-person's terms
- Counseling for family because just being able to talk to someone about what was happening would have helped. Information on support groups and meeting other families who have experienced such trauma, would have been extremely soothing
- Someone offering assistance with a list of attorneys, if needed, or other medical facilities better equipped and able to help patient progress
- Someone who would have been able to structure a program that would have fit my family's needs, for example, phone numbers of groups or organizations that offer help, and if out of town, assistance with lodging, meals, churches, etc.

After reading and realizing the lack of professional help my family had, I have to wonder what really helped us get through this experience. It seemed that everything that was needed by the family, the family provided. I thank God for giving us the strength, courage, and wisdom to endure each day and for watching over us as we struggle through head injury.

HIS MOTHER'S PERSPECTIVE

I remember lying in bed the night we got the phone call. I was wondering why Chris was late. It was 10:30 p.m. He had gone school shopping at the mall with a friend. It wasn't like him not to call if he was going to stop somewhere else.

Just the weekend before, he had finished up a grueling summer baseball schedule, playing 80-odd games in six weeks. He had worked so hard on getting a scholarship, and we were very proud of him. I remember his last tournament game. When they lost, he quickly tossed his uniform, like only a ball player could, to get ready for the drive to Walsh University where he would be attending in the fall. It was orientation weekend, but he had come back to play his final game. His dad had said, "Well, Chris, that was your last game." A strange feeling passed through me, and I quickly added, "Until you get to college." As we later drove to the hospital that night, that conversation kept floating through my thoughts.

We really didn't know how bad things were until we arrived at the hospital. When they told us he was having seizures and would need immediate brain surgery, we were devastated. Some friends of ours had gone through a similar experience just the year before, so were all too aware of the seriousness of the situation. As friends and family gathered at the hospital to keep a constant vigil, the pain and devastation set in. So many questions kept going through our minds. Would he live? If he did, how would he be? Why was this happening to us? The nurses were very helpful and brought much-needed comfort during the long weeks while he was in a coma. My husband and I could not bear to leave the hospital. The doctors did not seem to be educated enough to deal with the situation, so we finally had to make the agonizing decision to have him moved. All along we prayed to God to give us the strength, courage, and wisdom to make the right decisions.

My husband was offered a job, and the decision was made for him to go to work as I stayed with Chris. My husband quickly took over all the responsibilities of working and running the household, plus handling all the stacks of paperwork. I, on the other hand, was learning, right along with Chris, about therapy. Together we struggled to help him get better. For him, it was a matter of working relentlessly to make his body do what he wanted it to do. For me, it was the anguish of watching and being there for my child, but not really being able make it all better. It was a feeling of helplessness. I was determined to learn everything I could about head injury. Somehow being more knowledgeable on the subject made me feel more in control. I always tried to keep a cheerful, encouraging face on for Chris even though my heart was breaking. My other two sons were great. The middle son remained at home with his father and did everything he could to help out. My oldest son visited Chris daily and opened his bachelor apartment, which he was sharing with two other guys, to me.

Although the outlook was bleak, we never gave up hope that Chris would return to normal. But as we've learned, nothing is ever normal. Our lives are constantly changing. As Chris begins to have more and more control over his body, he seems more content. When Chris started school again after his injury I never imagined he would do this well or go this far. Having him transferred so far from home has been hard on the whole family, but he seems so happy that it's hard not to be happy for him. From the beginning, he was always accepted for who he was, not for what his body had trapped him into. The son we had was taken from us, but the son we were given back is even better in so many ways. Chris is a constant inspiration to all who come in contact with him. There is not a doubt in my mind that he will succeed in life.

As I reflect back, the pain and hurt will never go away, but I developed a tolerance for it. Life for all of us in this world is a challenge. You draw strength to meet those challenges through those around you. Things are so unpredictable, but would we really want to know how things will turn out? All we can hope for is to be surrounded by love, and the courage to face what life has to offer. A Garth Brooks song better explains this point: "Yes my life is better left to chance. I could have missed the pain, but I'd had to miss the dance."

Epilogue

Today Chris is working, married, and has three children, and that has made it all worthwhile.

DISCUSSION QUESTIONS

1. If you were engaged and your fiancée had a traumatic brain injury, what would you do? What would your family suggest?
2. How would you respond if you or a family member were brain injured as a result of violence?
3. Discuss the athletic frame of reference that Chris had and how it was an asset in treatment, recovery, and rehabilitation.
4. Why was Chris's family able to rally in a time of crisis?
5. If your loved one were not expected to survive, what would you do if faced with the decision concerning the use of life supports?
6. After reading this personal statement, would you consider rehabilitation at any cost?

7. What did Chris mean when he stated, "I know I gave it my best."
8. How can people learn to adapt to change as Chris and his family did?

SET 12: WHO NEEDS THIS KIND OF HELP?

When families are in a state of crisis, they need to be listened to, responded to, and treated with sensitivity, caring and respect. Often the stress of health care and rehabilitation environments creates a situation in which professional and nonprofessional staff do not provide help but rather create pain by insensitive and nonhelpful remarks.

Give two or three examples from your personal and/or professional frame of reference of how health care and human service professionals, as well as family and friends, have been helpful or unhelpful in dealing with the impact of an illness, disability, or loss.

Helpful responses:

1.
2.
3.

Unhelpful Responses:

1.
2.
3.

From your frame of reference what are the conditions and responses that would inspire hope, motivation, and coping if your family were faced with any of the situations presented in the personal statements in this book?

REFERENCES

Agency for Health Care Policy and Research (1998). Rehabilitation for Traumatic Brain Injury. Summary, Evidence Report/Technology Assessment, December 2, Portland, Oregon.

Blaylock, B. (2000). Patients' families as teachers: Inspiring an empathic connection. *Families, Systems, & Health, 18,*2, 161–175.

Callahan, D. (1987). *Setting limits: Medical goals in an aging society.* New York: Touchstone.

Callahan, D. (1999). *False hopes: Overcoming the obstacles to a sustainable, affordable medicine.* New Brunswick, NJ: Rutgers University Press.

Carroll, S. (1993). Spirituality and purpose in life in alcoholism recovery. *Journal of Studies on Alcohol,* May, 297-301.

Carson, V.B. (1993, Winter). Spirituality: generic or christian? *Journal of Christian Nursing,* 24-27.

Dell Orto, A. E., & Power, P. W. (2000). *Brain Injury and the Family.* Boca Raton, FL: CRC Press.

Gottschalk, L. A. (1985). Hope and other deterrents to illness. *American Journal of Psychotherapy,* 39, 515-524.

Halstead, L. S. (2001). The power of compassion and caring in rehabilitation healing. *Archives of Physical Medicine and Rehabilitation, 82,* February 2001, 149-154.

Herbert, J. (2003). Recovery and the rehabilitation process: A personal journey. *Rehabilitation Education, 17* (2), 125-132.

Kazak , A. E. (2002). Challenges in family health intervention research. *Family Systems & Health, 20*(1), 51-59.

Kay, J., & Raghavan, S. K. (2002). Spirituality in disability and illness. *Journal of Religion and Health, 41*(3), 231-242.

Koestenbaum, R.J. (1977). Death and development through the life span. In H. Feifel, *New meanings of death.* New York: McGraw-Hill.

Magaletta, P. R., & Oliver, J. M. (1999). The hope construct, wills and ways: Their relations with self-efficacy, optimism, and general well being. *Journal of Clinical Psychology, 55*(5), 539-551.

McColl, M. A., Bickenbach, J., Johnston, J., Nishihanma, S., Schumaker, M., Smith, K., Smith, M., & Yealland, B., (2000). Changes in spiritual beliefs after traumatic disability. *Archives of Physical Medicine and Rehabilitation, 81*(6), 817-823.

Miller, W. R., & Thoresen, C. E. (2003). Spirituality, religion and health: An emerging research field. *American Psychologist, 58*(1), 24-35.

New York Times (June 2003). *Improving the odds of good care,* p. A-22.

Nunn, K. (1996). Personal hopefulness: A conceptual review of the relevance of the perceived future to psychiatry. *British Journal of Medical Psychology, 69,* 227-245.

Phipps, E. J. (1998). Communication and ethics: Cardiopulmonary resuscitation in head trauma rehabilitation. *Journal of Head Trauma Rehabilitation,*13(5), 95-98.

Powell, L., Shahabi, L., & Thoresen, C. (2003). Religion and spirituality. *American Psychologist, 58*(1), 36-52.

Power, P. W., Dell Orto, A. E., & Gibbons, M. (1988). *Family interventions throughout chronic illness and disability.* New York: Springer Publishing.

Reed, P.G. (1991). Toward a nursing theory of self-transcendence: Deductive re-formulation using developmental theories. *Advances in Nursing Science,* 13 (4), 64-77.

Seeman,T. E., Fagan-Dubin, L., & Seemen, M.(2003). Religiosity/spirituality and health. *American Psychologist, 58*(1), 53-63.

Scheier, M. F. & Carver, C. S. (1992). Effects of optimism or psychological and physical well being: Theoretical overview and empirical update. *Cognitive Therapy and Research, 16,* 201-228.

Snyder, C. R., Irving, L. M., & Anderson, J. (1991). Hope and health. In C. R. Snyder & D. R. Forsyth (Eds.), *Handbook of Social and Clinical Psychology*. Elmsford, NY: Pergamon Press.

Weihs, K., Fisher, L, & Baird, M. (2002). Families, health, and behavior: A section of the commissioned report by the Committee on Health and Behavior: Research, practice, and policy. *Families, Systems & Health, 20*(1), 7–46.

Williams, G. C., Frankel, R. M., Campbell, T. L., & Deci, E. L.(2000). Research on relationship-centered care and health outcomes from the Rochester biopsychosocial program: A self-determination theory integration. *Family, Systems & Health, 18*(1), 79–90.

Young, C. (1993). Spirituality and the chronically ill Christian elderly. *Geriatric Nursing,* 14 (6), 298–303.

Author Index

Subject Index